THE BARTLETT POCKET GUIDE TO HIV/AIDS TREATMENT

2019

John G. Bartlett, M.D.
Professor Emeritus
Johns Hopkins University School of Medicine

Paul A. Pham, Pharm.D. BCPS
Managing Partner
Westview Urgent Care MediCenter
Adjunct Instructor of Medicine
Johns Hopkins University School of Medicine

Maunank Shah, M.D. Ph.D.
Associate Professor of Medicine
Johns Hopkins University School of Medicine

Important Information for the Users of This Pocket Guide

This document is provided as an information resource for physicians and other health care professionals to assist in the appropriate treatment of patients with HIV/AIDS. Recommendations for care and treatment change rapidly, and opinion can be controversial; therefore, physicians and other health care professionals are encouraged to consult other sources, especially FDA approved manufacturers' package inserts, and confirm the information contained on these tables. The individual health care professional should use his/her best medical judgment in determining appropriate patient care or treatment because no reference or guideline can trump provider judgment, based on individual patient issues, available resources, and updated information.

This pocket guide includes tables reflecting the authors' efforts to accurately report contemporary recommendation based largely on federal guidelines for HIV care and new developments by attendance at major scientific conferences and by systematic review of 42 relevant journals. Recommendations presented here are based largely on US federal guidelines for antiretroviral therapy for adults, pregnancy, prophylaxis and treatment of opportunistic infections, management of occupational exposure, management of co-infection with tuberculosis, hepatitis B, and hepatitis C, prevention of transmission, and management of sexually transmitted infections. Based on recent advances there has been substantial change in nearly all categories of care.

Inquiries, comments, and corrections about the Pocket Guide may be addressed to jgbartletthivguide@gmail.com

References for the HIV/AIDS Guide

Primary Care: Primary Care Guidelines for the Management of Persons Infected with Human Immunodeficiency Virus: 2013 Update by the HIV Medicine Association of the Infectious Diseases Society of America. Aberg JA, et al. Clin Infect Dis 2014; 58:1-10.

Antiretroviral Agents for Adults (DHHS): 2018 Guidelines for the Use of Antiretroviral Agents in HIV-1-Infected Adults and Adolescents, October 25, 2018. Available at http://www.aidsinfo.nih.gov/guidelines/.

WHO Guidelines: See Consolidated guidelines on HIV prevention, diagnosis, treatment and care for key populations, July 2016 (http://www.who.int/hiv/pub/guidelines/keypopulations-2016/en/)

Lipid Guidelines: 2013 ACC/AHA guideline on the assessment of cardiovascular risk: A report of the American College of Cardiology/American Heart Association Task Force on Practice Guideline. Stone NJ et al. Circulation 2014; 129 Suppl 2: S1-45

Antiretroviral Agents in Pregnancy 2018 DHHS: Recommendations for Use of Antiretroviral Drugs in Pregnant HIV-1-Infected Women for Maternal Health and Interventions to Reduce Perinatal HIV Transmission in the United States. May 30 2018. https://aidsinfo.nih.gov/guidelines/html/3/perinatal-guidelines/0/#

Prevention and treatment of Opportunistic Infections: DHHS Guidelines for the Prevention and Treatment of Opportunistic Infections in HIV-Infected Adults and Adolescents. Nov. 13th, 2018. https://aidsinfo.nih.gov/guidelines/html/4/adult-and-adolescent-oi-prevention-and-treatment-guidelines/0

TB Prevention and Treatment: TB Guidelines for HIV/TB co-infection: CDC guidelines 2013 www.cdc.gov/tb/publications/guidelines/Treatment.htm. American Thoracic Society / CDC/IDSA Treatment of Tuberculosis. MMWR 2005;54 (RR-12):1-81;(RR-15):1-47; and (RR-17):1-14:4-44); MMWR 2009;58(RR-4:1-207) and (RR-5:1-207); MMWR 2010;59 (RR-5):1-25. Available at http://www.cdc.gov/tb/. see DHHS Opportunistic Infection Guidelines-July 6, 2017 edition

STD Prevention and Treatment: Sexually Transmitted Disease Treatment CDC 2015 Guidelines. CDC MMWR Recomm and Rep 2015; 64: 1-137. Available at http://www.cdc.gov/std/tg2015/tg-2015-print.pdf

HIV Prophylaxis with Occupational HIV Exposure: Updated U.S. Public Health Service Guidelines for the Management of Occupational Exposures to HIV and Recommendations for Postexposure Prophylaxis - see: PEP Quick Guide for Occupational Exposures, CDC; Kuhar DT Infect Control Epidemiol 2013; 34: 875-92http://nccc.ucsf.edu/clinical-resources/pep-resources/pep-quick-guide/ updated 6/26/2017

Updated guidelines for antiretroviral postexposure prophylaxis after sexual, injection drug use, or other nonoccupational exposure to HIV—United States, 2016. https://stacks.cdc.gov/view/cdc/38856

HIV management with Encyclopedic Coverage: New York State AIDS Institute Guidelines. http://www.hivguidelines.org/

Pre-Exposure Prophylaxis (PrEP): CDC guidelines for the prevention of HIV infection in-2014. http://www.cdc.gov/hiv/pdf/prepguidelines2014.pdf

Antiretroviral Drug Resistance Mutation and Testing: 2018 Stanford database and 2018 Recommendations of IAS-USA. https://www.iasusa.org/sites/default/files/tam/24-4-132.pdfhttp://hivdb.stanford.edu.

Vaccines for HIV-infected persons: 2015 CDC Recommendations. Kim DK Ann Intern Med 2015; 162: 214-223. https://www.cdc.gov/mmwr/volumes/65/wr/mm6543a3.htm

HIV testing: 2015 CDC recommendations: Branson B. Curr HIV/AIDS Rep 2015;12:117-126

TABLE 1: Drug and Treatment Information Resources

Resource	Information and Source
AIDSInfo www.aidsinfo.nih.gov	DHHS Guidelines for ART in adults, pediatrics, and pregnancy
AETC www.aids-ed.org/aidsetc?page=cm-0D-0D	Clinical Manual for Management of the HIV-Infected Adult
AETC www.aids-ed.org	Training resources, slide sets, self study, and more
HIV InSite www.hivinsite.org	Knowledge base, drug interactions, global country profiles, and more
Johns Hopkins HIV Guide www.hopkins-hivguide.org	Clinical database, handheld HIV, publications, Q&A forum
Medscape HIV/AIDS www.medscape.com/hiv	News, conference coverage, drug interactions, reviews, Q&A, CME and more
National HIV/AIDS Clinicians Consultation Center www.nccc.ucsf.edu	AETC clinical resource, contact to warm line and PEPline
International AIDS Society-USA www.iasusa.org	CME, resistance mutation chart, cases
VA National HIV/AIDS Program www.hiv.va.gov	Information for providers and patients
International Training and Education Center on HIV www.go2itech.org	International AETC with training material
HIV Web Study depts.washington.edu/hivaids	University of Washington cases, tables, images
Stanford University HIV Drug Resistance Database hivdb.stanford.edu	Resistance mutations and interpretations
Clinical Care Options www.clinicaloptions.com/HIV.aspx	Reviews, CME, and conference summaries
New York State Department of Health AIDS Institute www.hivguidelines.org/	Guidelines for treatment of HIV, opportunistic infections, laboratory monitoring, systemic reviews, PEP, PrEP
Integrated services for HIV, STDs, hepatitis and TB for IDU pts (MMWR 2015; 65 (rr 13): 1-37)	HIV, STD, HBV, HCV, TB services
HIV Testing [Panner N, CDC: CID 2014; 59: 875-82; MMWR 2014; 63: 537] www.cdc.gov/mmwr/pdf/rr/rr5514.pdf	CDC recommendations for HIV screening 2014
Clinical Care Options http://www.clinicaloptions.com/HIV.aspx	News, conference coverage, drug interactions, reviews, Q&A, CME
HIV assist **https://www.hivassist.com/tool**	Interactive tool to assist clinicians in choosing the optimal ARV regimen based on patient specific variables: treatment history, resistance profile, and co-administered medications.

TABLE OF CONTENTS

TABLE 2: Abbreviations for Antiretroviral Agents and Classes

Antiretroviral Agents and Classes	
ABC: Abacavir (Ziagen)	InSTI: Integrase strand transfer inhibitor
ATV: Atazanavir (Reyataz)	LPV/r: Lopinavir/ritonavir (Kaletra)
AZT or ZDV: Zidovudine (Retrovir)	MVC: Maraviroc (Selzentry)
"/c": Boosted with cobicistat (Tybost)	NFV: Nelfinavir (Viracept)
COBI: Cobicistat (Tybost)	NNRTI: Non-nucleoside reverse transcriptase inhibitor
ddI: Didanosine (Videx)	NRTI: Nucleoside reverse transcriptase inhibitor
d4T: Stavudine (Zerit)	NVP: Nevirapine (Viramune)
DLV: Delavirdine (Rescriptor)	PI: Protease inhibitor
DTG: Dolutegravir (Tivicay)	PI/r: PI boosted with RTV
DOR: Doravirine (Pifeltro)	/r: Boosted with Ritonavir (RTV) $\leq$ 400 mg/d
DRV: Darunavir (Prezista)	RAL: Raltegravir (Isentress)
EFV: Efavirenz (Sustiva)	RPV: Rilpivirine (Edurant)
EVG: Elvitegravir (Vitekta)	RTV: Ritonavir (Norvir)
EI: Entry Inhibitor	SQV: Saquinavir (Invirase)
ENF: Enfuvirtide (Fuzeon, T-20)	3TC: Lamivudine (Epivir)
ETR: Etravirine (Intelence)	TAF: Tenofovir alafenamide
FPV: Fosamprenavir (Lexiva)	TDF: Tenofovir Disoproxil fumarate (Viread)
FTC: Emtricitabine (Emtriva)	TPV: Tipranavir (Aptivus)

Miscellaneous (cont.)

ACTG: AIDS Clinical Trial Group	ESRD: End-stage Renal Disease
ADR: Adverse Drug Reaction	ETOH: Alcohol
ART: Antiretroviral Therapy	FBS: Fasting Blood Glucose
AUC: Area Under the Concentration-Time Curve	FDA: US Food and Drug Administration
bid: twice per day	G6PD: Glucose 6-Phosphate Dehydrogenase
biw: twice per week	HAV: Hepatitis A Virus
BMD: Bone Mineral Density	HBsAb: Hepatitis B surface Antibody
CBC: Complete Blood Count	HBsAg: Hepatitis B surface Antigen
CDC: Centers for Disease Control	HBV: Hepatitis B Virus
CK: Creatine Kinase Assay	HCV: Hepatitis C Virus
CMV: Cytomegalovirus	HAART: Highly Active Antiretroviral Therapy
CPE: CNS penetration score	HIVAN: HIV-Associated Nephropathy
CPS: Child-Pugh Score	HIV-2: a retrovirus related to HIV
CrCl: Creatinine Kinase Clearance	HPV: Human Papilloma Virus
D/M tropic virus: Virus that is either dual-tropic (able to enter the CD4 cell using either the CCR5 or CXCR4 coreceptor) or a mixed population of R5- and X4-tropic virus	HSV-1: Herpes Simplex Virus Type 1
DEXA: Dual Energy X-ray	HSV-2: Herpes Simplex Virus Type 2
DHHS: US Department of Health and Human Services	hs: bedtime (hour of sleep)
DOT: Directly Observed Therapy	IDSA: Infectious Disease Society of America
DRESS: Drug Rash with Eosinophilia and Systemic Symptoms	IGRA: Interferon Gamma Releasing Assay
Dx: Diagnosis	IM: Intramuscular
EC: Enteric Coated	IRIS: Immune Reconstitution Inflammatory syndrome
EE: Ethinyl Estradiol	IV: Intravenous
EIA: Enzyme Immunoassay	IVIG: Intravenous Immune Globulin

TABLE 2: Abbreviations Used in This Pocket Guide (cont.)

Miscellaneous (cont.)

KS: Kaposi sarcoma	qid: four times per day
MAC: Mycobacterium avium complex	qm: monthly
MDRTB: Multidrug Resistant TB	qod: every other day
mo: month	qw: every week
MSM: Men who have sex with men	RAM: Resistance Associated Mutations
MTCT: Maternal to Child Transmission	R5 Tropic Virus: HIV strain that enters the CD4 cell using the CCR5 coreceptor
NAAT: Nucleic Acid Amplification Test	Rx: Treatment
nPEP: Non-Occupational Exposure Prophylaxis	SJS: Stevens-Johnson Syndrome
OI: Opportunistic Infection	soln: solution
PCP: Pneumocystis Pneumonia	std or SD: Standard (dose)
PCR: Polymerase Chain Reaction	STD: Sexually Transmitted Disease
PEP: Post-Exposure Prophylaxis	Sx: Symptoms
PGL: Peripheral Generalized Lymphadenopathy	TAM: Thymidine Analog Mutation
PML: Progressive Multifocal Leukoencephalopathy	TB: Tuberculosis
PrEP: Pre-Exposure Prophylaxis	TDM: Therapeutic Drug Monitoring
PI/c: Cobicistat-boosted Protease Inhibitor	TEN: Toxic Epidermal Necrolysis
PI/r: RTV boosted Protease Inhibitor	tid: three times per day
PML: Progressive Multifocal Leukoencephalopathy	tiw: three times per week
PMTCT: Prevention of Mother-To-Child Transmission	TMP/SMX: Trimethoprim + sulfamethoxazole
po: by mouth	ULN: Upper Limit of Normal
q: every	VL: Viral Load
qd: daily	VZIG: Varicella Zoster Immune Globulin
qid: four times per day	VZV: Varicella Zoster Virus
qm: monthly	X4-tropic Virus: HIV strains that enter the CD4 cell using the CXCR4 coreceptor

FORMULAS

TABLE 3A: Child-Pugh Score (CPS) for Hepatic Disease

Component	1 point	2 points	3 points
Encephalopathy	None	Gr 1-2	Gr 3-4
Ascites	None	Mild	Mod/Refractory
Albumin (g/dL)	> 3.5	2.8-3.5	< 2.8
Total bilirubin (mg/dL)	< 2	2-3	> 3
Pro-time sec. or INR	< 4 < 1.7	4-6 1.7-2.3	> 6 > 2.3

CP Classification
5-6 points: C-P A
7-9 points: C-P B
> 9 points: C-P C

Encephalopathy score
Gr 1: Mild confusion, fine tremor
Gr 2: Confusion, asterixis, disoriented
Gr 3: Somnolent, incontinence, incomprehensible
Gr 4: Coma, decerebrate posture, flaccid

TABLE 3B: Creatinine Clearance

Males:	$\dfrac{\text{Weight (kg) x (140-age)}}{72 \times \text{Serum creatinine (mg/dL)}}$
Females:	Value for males x 0.85
Note: Assumes stable renal function.	

TABLE 4: CDC HIV Staging System (MMWR 2014; 63 (RK03:1-10)

Stage	CD4	CD4%	Clinical
1	> 500	$\geq$ 26%	No AIDS-defining dx
2	200-499	14-25%	No AIDS-defining dx
3	< 200	< 14%	AIDS-defining dx

TABLE 5: AIDS-defining diagnoses

Definitions and frequency with CDC reported data for 1997 based on 23,527 US cases (last year the CDC collected and reported these data).

Candidiasis – esophagus, trachea, lungs – 16%

Cervical cancer, invasive – 0.6%

Coccidioidomycosis, extrapulmonary – 0.3%

Cryptococcosis, extrapulmonary – 5.0%

Cryptosporidiosis with diarrhea > 1 month – 1.3%

CMV – any organ but the liver, spleen, nodes (eye) – 7%

HSV with mucocutaneous ulcer > 1 month or bronchitis, pneumonia, esophagitis – 5%

Histoplasmosis, extrapulmonary – 0.9%

HIV dementia – disabling cognitive or other dysfunction interfering with normal function – 5%

Isosporoiasis with diarrhea > 1 month – 0.1%

Kaposi sarcoma – 7%

Lymphoma

   Burkitt – 0.7%

   immunoblastic – 2.3%

   primary CNS – 0.7%

M. avium or M. kansasii infection – extrapulmonary 5%

Tuberculosis

   pulmonary – 7%

   extrapulmonary – 2%

Pneumocystis pneumonia – 38%

Pneumonia, recurrent bacterial with > 2 episodes in 12 months – 5%

Progressive multifocal leukoencephalophy – 1%

Salmonellosis (nontyphoid), recurrent – 0.3%

Toxoplasmosis – internal organ – 4%

BASELINE EVALUATION
TABLE 6: Laboratory Tests
(DHHS ART Guidelines 2018; IDSA/HIVMA Primary Care Guidelines: Aberg J CID 2014; 58:1)

Test	Comment
HIV screening test	• 4th generation test (p24 Ag and HIV Ab) now preferred to detect early infection p24Ag and HIV antibody for HIV-1 and HIV-2. HIV testing algorithm (http://stacks.cdc.gov/view/cdc/48472). • Sensitivity and specificity standard serology is > 99% False positives: Usually human error False negatives: Usually 'window period' (uncommon with 4th gen test)
CD4 count and CD4 %	• Reproducibility: 95% CI: 30% • False high levels - splenectomy (use CD4%) or concurrent HTLV-1 (serologic test) • Repeat q3-6 mos; prior to ART, and during first 2 years of ART, during viremia, if receiving ART or if CD4 < 300/mm^3 • Repeat q12 month if on ART $\geq$ 2years with suppression & CD4 300-500/mm^3. • CD8 count and CD4/CD8 ratio are unnecessary and increase costs of test. • CD4 monitoring optional if on ART $\geq$ 2 years with viral suppression and CD4 > 500/mm^3.
HIV viral load	• Test at diagnosis; before starting ART; q2-4 weeks after initiating ART; thereafter q4-8 weeks until VL undetectable; within 2-4 weeks after virologic failure; q3-4 months during the first 2 years of ART, q6 month after 2 years of ART with consistent VL suppression. • Reproducibility: 95% CI - 0.3 log$_{10}$ c/mL or 50%
Genotypic Resistance Test	• Genotypic resistance test at diagnosis and with virologic failure while on ART or within 4 wks of stopping ART. Order INSTI resistance test if failing INSTI based regimen, or concern for transmitted INSTI resistance • Test at initiation of ART in pregnant women; optional in others if resistance genotype done at diagnosis.
CBC	• Repeat every 3-6 mos; more frequently as indicated (AZT) and co-morbidities • Repeat with treatment initiation or change. • Macrocytosis with AZT and d4T
Chemistry Profile (CMP, Creatinine, BUN, ALT, AST, Alk phos)	• Baseline, before and 2-8wks after ART initiation;repeat q6-12 mo • Repeat LFT q3-6 mos on ART and as clinically indicated • Repeat renal function with IDV & TDF (and possibly ATV and cobicistat) q3-6 mos • Serum Phos if CKD and on TDF or TAF
Hepatitis Screen: Anti-HAV, Anti-HCV, Anti-HBsAg, Anti-HBcAg, and HBsAg	• Standard screen: anti-HCV, anti-HAV, HBsAg, HBsAb, and anti-HBc • Repeat HBV screen prior to HCV treatment;Repeat HCV screen annually if at risk • Abnormal LFT: anti-HCV & HBsAg • Neg anti-HCV: not infected. Check HCV VL in pts at risk (e.g. IVDU) • Positive anti-HCV:check quantitative HCV RNA and HCV genotype • Positive HBsAg indicates acute or chronic: order HBV DNA, antiHBc, HBeAg • If HBsAg pos: treat HIV/HBV with TDF or TAF AND 3TC or FTC as NRTI backbone. • If anti-HBc positive but HBsAb negative, order HBV DNA. If negative, vaccinate • If HBsAg and HBsAb are negative: give HBV vaccine • Negative anti-HAV: HAV vaccine if risks (MSM, IDU, travelers) or consider in all non-immune pts; Positive anti-HAV: immune
Fasting lipid Profile:	• Assess cardiovascular risk. Test lipids at entry to care, at initiation of ART, then annually if normal or 4-8 weeks after starting or changing ART that affects lipids, then q6 mo if abnormal last test or if clinically indicated.
FBS and Hgb A1c	• FBS: Entry to care, prior to ART, q3-6 mo if last test abnormal or annually.

(continued)

Test	Comment
Toxoplasma IgG	• 10-30% positive in US; 50-80% in developing countries • If negative repeat if suspicion of toxoplasmosis (cannot be used to confirm or exclude Dx) or when CD4< 100/mm^3
PPD or Interferon Gamma Release Assay (IGRA)	• Screen at baseline; Repeat with new TB exposures; • IGRA or PPD can be used; IGRA advantages: more specific, one clinic visit, no BCG false positive, but increased cost. • Both tests may be false negative with advanced HIV;Repeat testing once CD4>200 if initial test negative • Induration > 5 mm or + IGRA is indication of TB infection (latent or active). If low exposure risk consider repeat testing • Chest X-ray to r/o active TB before latent TB treatment
Pap smear	• Baseline, at 6 mos, and then annual; if 'inadequate' repeat; if atypia - refer to gynecologist • HIVMA/IDSA HIV Primary care guidelines:anal pap tests for at risk MSM (anal receptive intercourse) and women with history of anal sex or abnormal cervical Paps; all with history of gential warts.
Urinary NAAT for N. gonorrhoeae, Chlamydia trachomatis and Trichomoniasis	• All women should be screened for trichomoniasis • Women < 25 yrs should be screened for C. trachomatis • Consider: in sexually active patients (see Table 53) • Repeat at 6-12 mos intervals depending on risk
HLA B*5701	• Screening before ABC treatment; negative test virtually excludes risk of ABC hypersensitivity reaction
Tropism Assay	• Screening before use of MVC. • R-5-tropic virus present in approximately 80% of treatment-naive patients vs. 40-60% in treatment-experienced.
Syphilis screening: Direct Treponemal Enzyme Immunoassay, then reflex to Non-treponemal tests (RPR)	• Baseline screening; annually if sexually active; more frequently based on risk. False positive RPR and low sensitivity in early primary and treated infections • LP if reactive serology and neuro or ocular symptoms • Traditional: RPR, then treponemal test if RPR+ • Some labs do reverse testing: Direct Treponemal test first, followed by RPR. • Positive EIA with negative RPR, requires confirmation with Treponema pallidum particle agglutination (TP-PA)
Renal Screen (urinalysis, Scr)	• Urinalysis and creatinine; entry to care, initiation of ART, repeat annually, q6 mo if underlying renal disease or on TDF or TAF. • If > 1+ proteinuria or elevated creatinine: quantify urine protein and order renal ultrasound if HIVAN suspected • Urine glucose and protein before starting TDF or TAF and monitor during treatment.
G6PD Level	• Recommended at baseline with predisposing background: most susceptible are men of African, Mediterranean, Asian, or Sephardic Jewish descent. Rate in African-American -10%, Hispanics - 2%, Caucasians - 0.7% (JID 2010;61:399) • If pos, avoid oxidant drugs dapsone and primaquine; ? sulfonamides. Rate of significant hemolysis with positive G6PD + TMP/SMX reported at 7% (JID 2010;61:399)

(continued)

TABLE 6: Laboratory Tests (cont.)

Test	Comment
Chest X-Ray	• Recommended for patients with pulmonary symptoms, history of a chronic chest disease or positive screening test for TB
CMV IgG; VZV IgG	• Identifies chronic infection. • Diagnostic: Consider CMV IgG in patients at low risk for CMV • VZV IgG recommended in those who don't recall history of chickenpox or shingles.
Testosterone	• Consider in men with fatigue, weight loss, decreased libido, erectile dysfunction, depression or osteoporosis • Obtain morning free serum testosterone
General Health Screens (Recommendations of US Public Service Task Force)	
Mammography	Biennial for women 50-74 yrs; optional age 40-49 (USPSTF2015)
Prostate Specific Antigen (PSA)	Recommended by American Cancer Society, but not USPSTF. Discuss pros and cons with patient.
Colorectal Cancer screening	Test occult blood, sigmoidoscopy, or colonoscopy age 50-75 years (USPSTF 2008)
Bone Densitometry	Recommended based on osteoporosis or FRAX score • National Osteoporosis Foundation: Women > 65 yrs, fragility fracture or persons > 50 yrs with risk (not including HIV) • HIVMA/IDSA HIV Primary Care Guidelines (CID 2014; 58:1): All HIV positive post-menopausal women and men > 50 yrs and all with fragility fractures

TABLE 7: Laboratory Monitoring Before and During ART

(DHHS Guidelines 2018)*

Test	Baseline	Before ART	ART Initiation	wk 2-8 follow-up	Every 3-6 Mo	Every 6-12 Mo	Viral Failure or clinically indicated
CD4	+	q3-6 mos	+		+ (first 2 years of ART; viremia on ART; CD4<300)	+ After 2 years of ART with VL <50 with CD4 300-500 q12 mos; Optional if VL < 50 and CD4 >500	+
Viral Load	+	optional	+	If VL >200	If VL <200	Every 6 months	+
Genotypic Resistance Test	+		+				+
Hepatitis B and C serology	+		+ (Hep B if neg at baseline)				+ (if starting HCV DAA)
Basic Chemistry	+	q6-12 mos	+	+	+		+
AST, ALT, Total Bilirubin	+	q6-12 mos	+	+	+		+
Beta-HCG	+		+				

* Repeat testing if clinically indicated

TABLE 7: Laboratory Monitoring Before and During ART (cont.)

Test	Baseline	Before ART	ART Initiation	wk 2-8 follow-up	Every 3-6 Mo	Every 6-12 Mo	Viral Failure or clinically indicated
CBC	+	q3-6 mos	+	+ (AZT)	+ (AZT)	+	+
Lipids/ FBS or A1C	+	Annual	+	*	*	+	+
Urinalysis	+		+	q6 mos with TAF orTDF		+	+

* Repeat testing if clinically indicated

TABLE 8: CD4 Cell Count   Correlation between CD4 count and CD4%:

CD4 Count	CD4%
> 500 cells/mm³	> 28%
200-500 cells/mm³	14-28%
< 200 cells/mm³	< 14%

Normal levels: 800-1050 cells/mm³ (95% CI=500-1400 cells/mm³)

Reproducibility: Approximately 30% for 2 SD; thus, a CD4 count of 200 could be reported at 118-337 cells/mm³

Deceptively high counts: Splenectomy or HTLV-1 infection

CD4%: Less variable metric

Recommendations for CD4 count testing (DHHS 2018): Entry to care, q3-6 months prior to ART, q3-6 months first 2 years of ART, or if viremia during ART or if CD4 count <200;

With VL suppression on ART and CD4 300-500: q12 months; CD4 > 500 and VL suppression: CD4 count monitoring is optional.

Expected CD4 response to ART:

Time	cells/mm³
4-8 weeks	+50
1 year	+100-150
5 years	+20-50/year

TABLE 9: Viral Load

Reproducibility: 2 SD = 3-fold or 0.5 $\log_{10}$ c/mL; thus, 95% CI for a VL of 10,000 c/mL would be 3,100-32,000 c/mL

Recommendations for Viral Load testing (DHHS Guidelines 2018): Entry to care; initiation of ART; if HIV RNA detectable at 2-8 weeks, repeat q4-8 wks until VL <200, then q3-4 months for first 2 yrs. If suppressed>2yrs and CD4>500, can extend to q6mo

Expected VL response to ART:

Treatment	VL ($\log_{10}$/mL)*
1 week	Decrease 0.75-1.0
4 weeks	Decrease 1.5-2.0; <5000 c/mL
8-16 weeks	< 500 c/mL
24-48 weeks	< 20 c/mL

* more rapid virologic response observed with InSTI-based regimens

TABLE 10: ARV formulations, dosing, and ADRs

Formulations(s)	Brand	Pill	Usual adult dose	Adverse Events
Once-Daily Co-Formulated ARV Regimens				
Bictegravir 50 mg/ Tenofovir alafenamide 25mg/ Emtricitabine 200mg tablet	Biktarvy		One tablet once-daily with food or without food.	-Generally well tolerated in clinical trials. -Less nausea compared to DTG/ABC/3TC -TAF: lower rates of nephrotoxicity than TDF, but avoid with CrCL <30ml/min. -TAF: possible HBV flare with discontinuation -TAF: lower rates of BMD loss than TDF -FTC: skin hyperpigmentation
Dolutegravir/ abacavir/ lamivudine* (DTG/ABC/3TC) 50/600/300 mg tablet	Triumeq		One tablet once-daily with or without food.	-Generally well tolerated in clinical trials with less discontinuation than with comparator ARVs (EFV, DRV/r) -DTG hypersensitivity reaction including rash, constitutional symptoms, and liver injury (rare). -Abacavir hypersensitivity reaction in HLA B*5701 positive pts (must pre-screen with HLA B*5701). -Possible HBV flare with 3TC discontinuation -Insomnia; headache -CK elevation -DTG: Serum creatinine elevation (no change in true GFR) -ABC: Possible increased risk of MI (controversial)
Dolutegravir 50mg/Rilpivirine 25 mg tablet	Juluca		One tablet once-daily with food.	-Use only as a simplification regimen in virologically suppressed pts with no resistance mutations to DTG or RPV. -Generally well tolerated in clinical trials -DTG hypersensitivity reaction including rash, constitutional syndrome, and liver injury (rare) -DTG: CK elevation -DTG: serum creatinine elevation (no change in true GFR -RPV: Dose dependent QTc prolongation; monitor QTc closely with PI/r, COBI, and other CYP3A inhibitor -RPV: Absorption dependent on food and gastric acid (avoid PPIs)
Elvitegravir/ cobicistat/ tenofovir DF alafenamide/ emtricitabine* (EVG/COBI/TAF/ FTC) 150/150/10/ 200 mg tablet	Genvoya		One tablet once-daily with food.	Generally well tolerated TAF: lower rates of nephrotoxicity than TDF, but do not use with CrCL <30 ml/min GI intolerance: nausea, diarrhea TAF/FTC: possible HBV flare with discontinuation TAF: lower rates of BMD loss than TDF FTC: skin hyperpigmentation
Elvitegravir/ cobicistat/ tenofovir DF/ emtricitabine* (EVG/COBI/TDF/ FTC) 150/150/300/ 200 mg tablet	Stribild		One tablet once-daily with food.	-Generally well tolerated with numerically lower discontinuation rates compared to EFV/TDF/FTC and ATV/r + TDF/FTC -TDF: nephrotoxicity (avoid in pts with CrCL <70 ml/min)-COBI: Serum creatinine elevation (no change in true GFR) -GI intolerance: nausea, diarrhea -TDF/FTC: Possible HBV flare with discontinuation -TDF: early loss of bone density -FTC: Skin hyperpigmentation.

*See Table 60 for dosing in renal failure

Formulations(s)	Brand	Pill	Usual adult dose	Adverse Events
Once-Daily Co-Formulated ARV Regimens				
Efavirenz/ tenofovir DF/ emtricitabine* (EFV/TDF/FTC) 600/300/200 mg tablet	Atripla		One tablet qhs without food. Can be taken with food or in the morning if tolerated	-EFV: Morbilliform rash in up to 26% of pts requiring discontinuation in 1.7% (median onset 11 days, duration 16 days) -EFV: Teratogenic in non-human primates, but can be used in pregnant patients after 8 week gestation -EFV: CNS side effects: vivid dreams including nightmares, nocturnal dizziness, morning confusion; depersonalization, possible suicidality (worse during the first 2 weeks, but can persist) -EFV: False positive THC and benzodiazepine screening test -EFV: Hyperlipidemia -EFV: Increased LFTs -TDF: nephrotoxicity -TDF: early loss of bone density -TDF/FTC: Possible HBV flare with discontinuation
Efavirenz/ tenofovir DF/ lamivudine* (EFV/TDF/3TC) 600/300/300 mg tablet	Symfi		Use Symfi tab for patients ≥ 40kg or higher.	
Efavirenz/ tenofovir DF/ lamivudine* (EFV/TDF/3TC) 400/300/300 mg tablet	Symfi Lo		Use Symfi Lo tab for patients ≥ 35kg (with CNS side effects on EFV 600mg)	
Rilpivirine/ tenofovir alafenamide/ emtricitabine* (RPV/TAF/FTC) 25/25/200 mg tablet	Odefsey		One tablet once-daily with food.	-Poorer performance with VL >100K and CD4 <200 -RPV: dose dependent QTc prolongation; monitor QTc with PI/r, COBI, and other CYP3A4 inhibitors -TAF: lower rates of nephrotoxicity than TDF, but do not use with CrCL <30 ml/min -GI intolerance: nausea, diarrhea -TAF/FTC: possible HBV flare with discontinuation -TAF: lower rates of BMD loss than TDF -FTC: skin hyperpigmentation
Rilpivirine/ tenofovir DF/ emtricitabine* (RPV/TDF/FTC) 25/300/200 mg tablet	Complera		One tablet once-daily with food. -RPV: Absorption dependent on food and gastric acid; must be taken with meal, and not with PPIs	-Better tolerated than EFV/TDF/FTC -Poorer performance with VL >100K and CD4 <200 -TDF: nephrotoxicity -TDF: early loss of bone density -TDF/FTC: Possible HBV flare with discontinuation -RPV: Dose dependent QTc prolongation; monitor QTc closely with PI/r, COBI, and other CYP3A inhibitors. -RPV: resistance with 138K mutation leads to etravirine cross-resistance
Doravirine/ tenofovir DF/ lamivudine* (DOR/TDF/3TC) 100/300/300 mg tablet	Delstrigo		One tablet once-daily with or without food	-Generally well tolerated -Less CNS side effects compared to EFV -TDF: nephrotoxicity -TDF: early loss of bone density -TDF/FTC: Possible HBV flare with discontinuation

*See Table 60 for dosing in renal failure

TABLE 10: ARV formulations, dosing, and ADRs (cont.)

Formulations(s)	Brand	Pill	Usual adult dose	Adverse Events
Co-Formulated nucleoside reverse transcriptase inhibitors (NRTIs)				
Zidovudine/ abacavir/ lamivudine* (AZT/ABC/3TC) 300/300/150 mg tablet	Trizivir; generic		One tablet twice-daily with or without food.	-ABC hypersensitivity reaction in HLA B*5701 positive pts (must pre-screen with HLA B*5701). -AZT: GI intolerance: nausea, vomiting -AZT: Headache, asthenia -AZT: Bone marrow suppression (macrocytic anemia, neutropenia) -AZT: Mitochondrial toxicity with (lactic acidosis, hepatic steatosis)-must discontinue -AZT: Lipoatrophy, myopathy -ABC: Possible increased risk of MI (controversial) -3TC: Possible HBV flare with 3TC discontinuation
Tenofovir alafenamide /emtricitabine* (TAF/FTC) 25/200 mg tablet	Descovy		One tablet once-daily with or without food	-Generally well tolerated -Lower rates of nephrotoxicity than TDF -Lower rates of BMD Loss than TDF -GI intolerance and nausea -Possible HBV flare with TAF/FTC discontinuation
Tenofovir DF/ emtricitabine* (TDF/FTC) 300/200 mg tablet	Truvada		One tablet once-daily with or without food	-Generally well tolerated -TDF: GI intolerance: nausea, vomiting, diarrhea, flatulence -TDF: Nephrotoxicity, including proximal tubular dysfunction -TDF/FTC: Possible HBV flare with TDF/FTC discontinuation -TDF: Early loss of bone density. -TDF: Headache
Tenofovir DF/ lamivudine* (TDF/3TC) 300/300 mg tablet	Cimduo		One tablet once-daily with or without food	-Generally well tolerated -TDF: GI intolerance: nausea, vomiting, diarrhea, flatulence -TDF: Nephrotoxicity, including proximal tubular dysfunction -TDF/3TC: Possible HBV flare with TDF/3TC discontinuation -TDF: Early loss of bone density. -TDF: Headache
Zidovudine/ lamivudine• (AZT/3TC) 300/150 mg tablet	Combivir; generic		One tablet twice-daily with or without food.	-AZT: GI intolerance: nausea, vomiting -AZT: Headache, asthenia -AZT: Bone marrow suppression (macrocytic anemia, neutropenia) -AZT: Mitochondrial toxicity (Lactic acidosis, hepatic steatosis)-must discontinue -AZT: Lipoatrophy, myopathy -AZT: Nail hyperpigmentation-3TC -Possible HBV flare with 3TC discontinuation
Abacavir/ lamivudine* (ABC/3TC) 600/300mg tablet	Epzicom		One tablet once-daily with or without food.	-Inferior VL response with VL >100K when combined with EFV or ATV/r, but not with DTG -ABC hypersensitivity reaction in HLA B*5701 positive pts (must prescreen with HLA B*5701). -ABC: Possible increased risk of MI (controversial) -TDF/FTC: Possible HBV flare with discontinuation

*See Table 60 for dosing in renal failure

TABLE 10: ARV formulations, dosing, and ADRs (cont.)

Formulations(s)	Brand	Pill	Usual adult dose	Adverse Events
Co-formulated boosted Protease Inhibitors (PI/cobi)				
Darunavir/ cobicistat (DRV/c) 800/150 mg tablet	Prezcobix		One tablet once-daily with food	-GI intolerance: nausea, vomiting, diarrhea -Rash (contains a sulfonamide moiety, but not contraindicated with sulfa allergy). Avoid with a history of severe sulfa allergy (eg SJS/TEN) -COBI: increase serum creatinine (no change in actual GFR).
Darunavir/ cobicistat/ Tenofovir Alafenamide/ Emtricitabine (DRV/c/TAF/FTC) 800/150/25/200 mg tablet	Symtuza		One tablet once-daily with food	-Hepatitis; Headache -TAF: lower rates of nephrotoxicity than TDF -TAF: lower rates of BMD Loss than TDF -GI intolerance and nausea -Possible HBV flare with TAF/FTC discontinuation
Atazanavir/ cobicistat (ATV/c) 300/150 mg Tablet	Evotaz		One tablet once-daily with food	-GI intolerance: nausea, vomiting, diarrhea -LFT elevation; Rash -ATV: Benign increase in indirect bilirubin, but may cause jaundice and/or scleral icterus -PR interval prolongation -COBI: Increase in serum creatine (no change in actual GFR) -ATV: Nephrotoxicity with or without nephrolithiasis (reported with ATV/r) -ATV: Cholelithiasis
Nucleoside reverse transcriptase inhibitors (NRTIs)				
Abacavir (ABC) 300 mg tablet 20 mg/ml solution	Ziagen, generic		600mg once-daily with or without food	-ABC hypersensitivity reaction in HLA B*5701 positive pts (must pre-screen with HLA B*5701). -Possible increased risk of MI (controversial) -Less effective at VL >100,000 when combined with EFV or ATV/r, but not DTG
Didanosine* (ddI) 125, 200, 250, 400 mg EC capsules 10 mg/mL solution	Videx. generic		>60kg: 400 mg once-daily <60kg: 250 mg once-daily With TDF: ddI 250 mg once-daily	-Mitochondrial toxicity (lactic acidosis, hepatic steatosis peripheral neuropathy and pancreatitis)-must discontinue -GI intolerance: nausea, vomiting -Possible increase in MI risk -Insulin resistance/DM; Possible non-cirrhotic portal -Not recommended
Emtricitabine* (FTC) 200 mg cap 10 mg/mL Soln	Emtriva		200mg once-daily	-Generally well tolerated -Possible HBV flare with discontinuation -Skin hyperpigmentation
Lamivudine* (3TC) 150 mg and 300 mg tablets 10 mg/mL soln.	Epivir, generic		300mg once daily or 150 mg twice-daily	-Generally well tolerated -Possible HBV flare in co-infected pts with 3TC discontinuation
Stavudine* (d4T) 15, 20,30, and 40 mg capsules 1mg/ml oral solution	Zerit, generic		40 mg twice daily (but associated with greater toxicity) 30 mg twice-daily	-Mitochondrial toxicity (lactic acidosis, hepatic steatosis peripheral neuropathy)-must discontinue -Lipoatrophy; -Hyperlipidemia -Progressive ascending neuromuscular weakness (rare)-must discontinue -Insulin resistance/DM
Tenofovir diproxil fumarate* (TDF) 150, 200, 250, 300 mg tablets 40 mg/g oral powder	Viread; generic		300 mg once-daily with or without food.	-Generally well tolerated -GI intolerance: nausea, vomiting, diarrhea, flatulence -Nephrotoxicity, including proximal tubular dysfunction -Early decrease in bone density -Possible HBV flare with discontinuation

*See Table 60 for dosing in renal failure

Formulations(s)	Brand	Pill	Usual adult dose	Adverse Events
Nucleoside reverse transcriptase inhibitors (NRTIs)				
Zidovudine* (AZT) 100 mg capsule 10 mg/mL oral solution 10 mg/mL IV solution Generic: 300mg tab	Retrovir, generic		300 mg twice-daily with or without food.	-GI intolerance: nausea, vomiting -Headache, asthenia -Bone marrow suppression (macrocytic anemia, neutropenia) -Mitochondrial toxicity (lactic acidosis, hepatic steatosis)-must discontinue -Lipoatrophy -Myopathy -Nail hyperpigmentation
Non-nucleoside reverse transcriptase inhibitors (NNRTIs)				
Etravirine (ETR) 25, 100 and 200mg tablets	Intelence		200mg twice daily with food. 400 mg once daily may be considered based on PK studies.	-Generally well tolerated -GI: nausea -Rash: generally mild to moderate (but SJS has been reported), occurs in 2nd wk and resolves within 1-2 wks on continued therapy. SJS has been reported. -HSR reaction: Rash, constitutional Sx, hepatitis; discontinue ETR.
Nevirapine (NVP) 200 mg tablet and 400mg XR tablet 50mg/5mL oral suspension	Viramune, generic		200 mg once daily x 2 wks then 200mg twice daily (OR 400 mg XR tab once daily) with or without food. Avoid initiating in men with pre-treatment CD4 >400 men women with CD4 >250.	-Rash is common (up to 50% of pts). Severe rashes including SJS and TEN more common compared to other NNRTIs -Severe hepatitis, including fatal hepatic necrosis (increased risk win women with CD4 >250 and men with CD4 >400 at initiation of therapy).
Rilpivirine (RPV) 25mg tablet	Edurant		25mg once daily with food. Food and acidic gastric pH critical for absorption. Avoid antacids, H2-blockers, PPIs	-Hepatitis -Dose dependent QTc prolongation; monitor with CYP3A4 inhibitors co-administration. -Depression (8%; most were mild or moderate in severity. The rate of Grade 3 or 4 depression was 1%) -Insomnia, headache
Doravirine (DOR) 100 mg tablet	Pifeltro		100 mg once daily with or w/o food	-Generally well tolerated -Less CNS side effects compared to EFV -GI: nausea, abd pain, diarrhea

*See Table 60 for dosing in renal failure

TABLE 10: ARV formulations, dosing, and ADRs (cont.)

Formulations(s)	Brand	Pill	Usual adult dose	Adverse Events
Protease Inhibitors (PIs)				
Atazanavir (ATV) 100, 150, 200, and 300 mg capsules 50 mg oral powder packet Generic: 150, 200, 300 mg cap.	Reyataz; generic		400 mg once daily OR 300 mg (plus ritonavir 100 mg or cobicistat 150 mg) once daily with food With EFV, use ATV 400 mg + RTV 100 mg. Avoid antacid, H-2 blocker, and PPIs or use with recommended dose separation.	-GI intolerance: nausea, vomiting, diarrhea -Hyperlipidemia with boosted ATV, but less common compared to older PIs. -Benign increase in indirect bilirubin; may cause jaundice or scleral icterus -PR interval prolongation including first degree block -Nephrotoxicity with or without nephrolithiasis -Cholelithiasis -Rash
Darunavir (DRV) 75, 150, 600 and 800mg tablets 100 mg/mL oral suspension	Prezista		800mg with ritonavir 100mg or cobicistat 150 mg once daily OR 600mg with ritonavir 100mg twice daily with food. Twice-daily dosing recommended in pts with DRV-associated mutations.	-GI intolerance: nausea, vomiting, diarrhea -Rash reported in 10% (contains a sulfonamide moiety, but not contraindicated in patents with sulfa allergy). Avoid with a history of severe sulfa allergy (eg JS/TEN) -Hepatitis -Headache
Fosamprenavir (FPV) 700mg tablet 50 mg/mL oral suspension	Lexiva		FPV/r 700/100 mg twice daily OR FPV/r 1400 /100 mg once daily (PI-naïve only) with or without food. FPV 1400 mg twice-daily (not recommended) With EFV co-administration, FPV/r 1400/300 mg once-daily OR FPV/r 700/100 mg twice-daily.	-GI intolerance: nausea, vomiting, diarrhea -Rash reported in 12-19% (contains a sulfonamide moiety). Avoid with a history of severe sulfa allergy (eg SJS/TEN) -Hepatitis -Headache -Nephrolithiasis (rare) -May increase risk of bleed in pts with hemophilia -Resistance (usually with unboosted FPV) can lead to DRV-cross-resistance -Not a recommended PI (DHHS guidelines)
Indinavir (IDV) 100, 200, 400 mg capsules	Crixivan		IDV 800 mg q8h 1 hr or 2 hrs after meals. IDV/r 800/100 mg twice-daily	-PI class ADR: Hyperglycemia, LFTs elevation, fat accumulation, hyperlipidemia -Asthenia, headache, metallic taste -GI intolerance: nausea, vomiting, diarrhea -Benign increase in indirect bilirubin; may cause jaundice or scleral icterus -May increase risk of bleed in pts with hemophilia -Nephrolithiasis, nephrotoxicity -Retinoid effects: paronychia, xerosis, hair loss

*See Table 60 for dosing in renal failure

TABLE 10: ARV formulations, dosing, and ADRs (cont.)

Formulations(s)	Brand	Pill	Usual adult dose	Adverse Events
Protease Inhibitors (PIs)				
Lopinavir/ritonavir (LPV/r) 200/50 mg and 100/25mg tablets 400/100 mg per 5 ml oral solution	Kaletra		LPV/r 400/100 twice daily OR LPV/r 800/100 mg once daily with or without food	-PI class ADR: Hyperglycemia, LFTs elevation, fat accumulation, hyperlipidemia -GI intolerance: nausea, vomiting, diarrhea (higher rates than ATV/r and DRV/r). -QTc and PR prolongation -May increase risk of bleed in pts with hemophilia -Asthenia -Pancreatitis
Nelfinavir (NFV) 250 mg and 625 mg tablets 50mg/g oral powder	Viracept		NFV 1250 mg twice daily with fatty meals OR NFV 750 mg three times a day with fatty meals.	-PI class ADR: Hyperglycemia, LFTs elevation, fat accumulation, hyperlipidemia -GI intolerance: nausea, vomiting, secretory diarrhea -May increase risk of bleed in pts with hemophilia -Inferior virologic suppression compared to other PIs and cannot be boosted: Not recommended
Saquinavir (SQV) 500 mg and 200 mg capsule	Invirase		SQV/r 1000/100 mg twice-daily.	-PI class ADR: Hyperglycemia, LFTs elevation, fat accumulation, hyperlipidemia -GI intolerance: nausea, vomiting, diarrhea -Hepatitis -QTc (avoid if QTc >450 ms); get baseline EKG -PR prolongation -May increase risk of bleed in pts with hemophilia
Tipranavir (TPV) 250mg capsulte 100 mg/mL oral solution	Aptivus	TPV 250	TPV/r 500/200mg twice-daily with food.	-PI class ADR: Hyperglycemia, LFTs elevation, fat accumulation, hyperlipidemia -GI intolerance: nausea, vomiting, diarrhea -Rash reported in 3-21% (contains a sulfonamide moiety). Avoid with a history of severe sulfa allergy (eg SJS/TEN) -May increase risk of bleed in pts with hemophilia -High incidence of hepatitis including fatalities -Intracranial hemorrhage (rare) -Recommended only for use in treatment experienced patients with virus that is resistant to other PIs but susceptible to TPV
Integrase Inhibitors (INSTI)				
Dolutegravir (DTG) 50mg tablet	Tivicay	50	50mg once-daily with or without food or 50 mg twice-daily with or without food if integrase mutations present. 50 mg twice-daily when combined with FPV/r, TPV/r, EFV.	-Generally well tolerated in clinical trials with more patients discontinuing comparator ARVs (EFV, DRV/r) -DTG hypersensitivity reaction including rash, constitutional symptoms, and liver injury (rare). -Insomnia, headache -CK elevation -Serum creatinine elevation without change in actual GFR
Raltegravir (RAL) 400 mg tablet 25 and 100 mg chewable tablets 100 mg per pack oral suspension	Isentress	227	400 mg twice-daily with or without food	-Generally well tolerated, with comparable ADR rates to placebo in clinical trials. -GI intolerance: nausea, diarrhea -CK elevation (rhabdomyolysis reported) -Headache, insomnia -Fever (unclear association) -Rash (rare cases of SJS, HSR, and TEN reported)
Raltegravir (RAL HD) 600mg tablet	Isentress HD		1200 mg (2x 600mg tab) once-daily with or without food (for treatment-naive pts)	

*See Table 60 for dosing in renal failure

TABLE 10: ARV formulations, dosing, and ADRs (cont.)

Formulations(s)	Brand	Pill	Usual adult dose	Adverse Events
Monoclonal Antibody				
Ibalizumab-uiyk 200 mg/1.33ml (150mg/ml) vial	Trogarzo		2000mg IV (over 30 mins) x1, then 800 mg IV (over 15mins) q2 weeks	Diarrhea, dizziness, nausea, rash (reported in heavily treatment experienced patients)
Entry Inhibitors (fusion inhibitor)				
Enfuvirtide (T20) 90 mg/mL vial	Fuzeon		90 mg (1mL) SC twice-daily	-Injection site reaction (e.g pain, erythema, induration) -cases of hypersensitivity reaction (rash, fever, chills, hepatitis, nausea, vomiting, and hypotension) do not rechallenge. -Possible increased risk of bacterial pneumonia
Entry Inhibitors (CCR5 blocker)				
Maraviroc* (MVC) 150 and 300mg tablets	Selzentry		-With all NRTIs, BIC, DTG, RAL, TPV/r, RPV, DOR (without PIs, COBI, EFV, or ETR): MVC 300 mg twice-daily Must pre-screen for R5 tropism	-Generally well tolerated in clinical trials, with similar rates of discontinuation vs. placebo -GI: diarrhea, nausea, abdominal pain -CK elevation, myalgia -Hepatotoxicity (preceded by severe rash and eosinophilia, elevated IgE) -Fever -Dizziness Dosing with CY3A4 inhibitors -With all PIs (except TPV/r) and COBI: MVC 150 mg twice-daily. Dosing with CY3A4 inducers -With EFV and ETR (without a PI): MVC 600 mg twice daily If RTV- or COBI-boosted regimen given with EFV or ETR: MVC 150 mg twice-daily.
Pharmacokinetic Enhancer/CYP3A4 inhibitor				
Cobicistat (COBI or /c) 150 mg tablet	Tybost		150 mg once daily with food in combination with with DRV 800 mg QD OR ATV 300 mg QD	-GI intolerance -Increased serum creatinine without effect on actual GFR
Ritonavir (RTV or /r) 100mg tablet 100 mg soft gel capsule 80mg/mL oral solution 100 mg oral powder packet	Norvir; generic		Pharmacokinetic enhancer (booster) of other PIs: 100 – 200mg once or twice a day. RTV 600 mg twice a day is not recommended.	-PI class ADR: Hyperglycemia, LFTs elevation, fat accumulation, hyperlipidemia -Dose dependent GI intolerance: nausea, vomiting, diarrhea -Dose dependent hepatitis -Circumoral paresthesia, asthenia, taste perversion associated with full dose RTV.

TABLE 11: Adverse Reactions of Antiretroviral Agents

Life Threatening Reactions	
Hepatic Necrosis	
Agent	NVP
ADR Features	Abrupt onset of flu-like illness with GI symptoms, fever, rash (50%), eosinophilia and hepatic necrosis usually in first 6 wks and up to 18 weeks.
Frequency	1-2% of all NVP recipients. Rate of symptomatic hepatitis is 11% in treatment-naive women with baseline CD4 count > 250 cells/mm^3 and 6% in men with baseline CD4 count > 400 cells/mm^3. No risk with single dose for PMTCT.
Monitor	Warn patient. ALT: Baseline and at 2 wks and 4 wks; then monthly x 3 mos, then q3mos.
Intervention	Promptly discontinue ART, but may progress despite this. Supportive care (steroids, antihistamines appear ineffective). Do not rechallenge. Safety of NNRTI switch unknown.
Cutaneous: Stevens-Johnson Syndrome and Toxic Epidermal Necrolysis	
Agent	NVP; less common with EFV, ETR, RPV (reported with FPV, DRV, TPV, ABC, ddI, LPV, AZT, ATV, RAL and IDV).
ADR Features	Usually first few weeks with fever, myalgia, skin rash with blistering ± mucous membrane; involvement with NVP may also cause hepatic necrosis.
Frequency	NVP 0.5-1%, EFV 0.1%, ETR < 0.1%; RPV (uncommon)
Monitor	Warn patient
Intervention	Promptly discontinue ART if mucous membrane involved, conjunctivitis, blisters, bullae, and/or system symptoms. Intensive care of wounds including pain meds and antibiotics and IVs; may require treatment in a burn center. Role of steroids and IVIG unclear.
Lactic Acidosis	
Agent	d4T > ddI > AZT (Rare or never with ABC, TDF, 3TC, and FTC); more common w/ long duration use.
ADR Features	GI symptoms, wasting, fatigue, ± multiorgan failure, pancreatitis, respiratory failure.
Frequency	1-10 per 1,000 patient-years for d4T or ddI. Risk: d4T > ddI > AZT; Female, obesity; dose and duration related.
Monitor	Clinical symptoms. No routine lactate levels, but obtain if clinically indicated; normal level is < 2.0 mmol/L. Surrogate for lactic acid levels: High CPK and ALT; low HCO$_3$; anion gap.
Intervention	Promptly discontinue ART; supportive care with mechanical ventilation, dialysis, HCO$_3$ infusion, hemofiltration. Role of steroids, carnitine, thiamine, IVIG, plasmapheresis, or riboflavin: unclear. Recovery may take months. Long-term residual effects are common. For ART avoid NRTI or use ABC, 3TC, FTC, and/or TDF. Case reports of benefit from L-carnitine, riboflavin.

Life Threatening Reactions (cont.)	
Hypersensitivity (HSR)	
Agent	Common: ABC; NVP Uncommon: RAL (DTG<1%); MVC
ADR Features	ABC Symptoms (in rank order): high fever, diffuse skin rash, nausea, headache, abdominal pain, diarrhea, arthralgias, pharyngitis, and dyspnea. Virtually all have ≥ 2 systems involved (may help distinguish common intercurrent illnesses). Always progresses with continued ABC use. Median onset: day 9 of ABC; 90% in first 6 wks. NVP: see hepatic necrosis RAL: severe rash including rash w/ eosinophilia and systemic symptoms MVC: see hepatitis
Frequency	ABC: 6-7% of ABC recipients; very rare or never if HLA-B* 5701 is negative. Risk lower in African-Americans. NVP: Up to 11% in women with CD4 > 250
Monitor	ABC: Warn patient. (In questionable cases, administer next dose under observation - this reaction always progresses with next dose). NVP: Monitor for rash, hepatitis, fever in first 6-8 weeks
Intervention	ABC: D/C ABC. Never re-challenge (if dx is likely). Supportive care (steroids and antihistamines are not useful). Symptoms usually resolve in 48 h after D/C ABC. NVP: D/C NVP ASAP
Serious Reactions	
Pancreatitis	
Agent	ddI + d4T > ddI > d4T
ADR Features	Abdominal pain with elevated amylase and/or lipase.
Frequency	ddI 1-7%. More frequent with other risk factors-especially alcoholism, hx pancreatitis, concurrent d4T, ddI and TDF without ddI dose adjustment, ddI + ribavirin (contraindicated).
Monitor	Warn patient. Amylase and lipase with clinical symptoms.
Intervention	Supportive care, pain meds and bowel rest (NPO).
Nephrotoxicity	
Agent	TDF+boosted ATV>TDF+PI/r>TDF>IDV>ATV (possibly LPV/r)>>TAF
ADR Features	TDF: Renal failure ± Proximal tubulopathy or full Fanconi syndrome. Note: increased creatinine, proteinuria, hypophosphotemia, renal phosphate wasting, glycosuria, hypokalemia, non-anion gap, metabolic acidosis. May be asymptomatic or signs of diabetes insipidus. Risks: Advanced age; low BMI, low CD4, concurrent use of PI/r or PI/c; avoid TDF with CrCl < 50 mL/min unless end-stage renal disease. ATV/IDV: nephrotoxicity +/- nephrolithiasis
Frequency	Low, but increase with long term use and possibly with boosted PI co-administration.
Monitor	Monitor urinalysis and Scr. If proteinuria or decreased CrCL then measure urine protein/creatinine or albumin/creatinine ratio
Intervention	Evaluate and use alternative agent. Switch from TDF to ABC or TAF (if CrCL >30 ml/min). Note: RPV, DTG, EVG/c, BIC, COBI inhibits tubular secretion of Scr but no change in GFR.

TABLE 11: Adverse Reactions of Antiretroviral Agents

Serious Reactions (cont.)	
Renal calculi	
Agent	IDV >> ATV
ADR Features	Renal colic, abdominal pain, hematuria. UA shows RBC, pyuria,and crystals.
Frequency	5-35%; correlates with high peak IDV blood level. ATV is uncommon cause.
Monitor	Urinalysis ± creatinine or BUN q3-5mos with IDV.
Intervention	Avoid or D/C IDV. Prevention is hydration with ≥ 1.5 L/d with IDV. Manage as nephrolithiasis. IDV should be stopped or given with better hydration.
Bone marrow suppression	
Agent	ZDV
ADR Features	Neutropenia and/or macrocytic anemia usually after weeks-months.
Frequency	Anemia 1-4%, neutropenia 2-8%. Risk increased with advanced HIV. ANC < 500 in 2-8%.
Monitor	CBC at baseline and q3mos for ZDV recipients.
Intervention	Avoid or D/C AZT. Transfusion or EPO for serious anemia; GCSF for neutropenia. D/C ZDV.
Hepatitis	
Agent	All PIs (TPV/r>>all other PIs), NNRTIs (NVP>>EFV>ETR, RPV, DOR), some NRTIs (d4T, ddI + AZT), and MVC, DTG. Note: Discontinuation or development of resistance to 3TC, FTC, TAF and TDF can cause HBV flare in HIV/HBV co-infection.
ADR Features	Elevated ALT that is otherwise not explained (ETOH, hepatitis B, hepatitis C etc). PI/NNRTI: mechanism is unknown. Liver biopsy usually does not show hepatic injury. Most are asymptomatic - exceptions are NVP-associated hepatic necrosis and NRTI-associated lactic acidosis (AZT, d4T, ddI) with steatosis. MVC hepatitis preceded by rash and increased IgE. ddI: non-cirrhotic portal hypertension
Frequency	8-15% for most PIs and NNRTIs.
Monitor	ALT q3-4mos
Intervention	Must distinguish ALT elevations due to other drugs (lactic acidosis with steatosis due to d4T, ddI or ZDV), from hypersensitivity due to ABC, or NVP hepatic necrosis) and other causes (hepatitis viruses, IRIS, ETOH, etc). Many D/C the PI or NNRTI if the ALT is > 5x ULN (Grade 3 toxicity) or 10x ULN (Grade 4), or if symptomatic or ↑ Bilirubin (Total) > 2x ULN with ALT > 3x ULN. Avoid EFV, NVP, TPV with Child-Pugh Class B or C

TABLE 11: Adverse Reactions of Antiretroviral Agents

Miscellaneous Reactions	
GI intolerance	
Agent	All PIs: LPV/r ≈ FPV/r > ATV/r, ATV/cobi, > DRV/r, DRV/cobi, SQV/r NRTIs: ZDV > ddI> other NRTIs EVG/COBI/TDF/FTC> DTG/ABC/3TC > BIC/TAF/FTC
ADR Features	Nausea, vomiting, diarrhea, anorexia. Begins with first dose. Diarrhea: LPV/r, NFV, buffered ddI
Frequency	Common
Monitor	Warn patient
Intervention	Symptomatic - may improve with food (except ddI and IDV without RTV); NFV and LPV/r-associated diarrhea is usually managed with loperamide, calcium; many improve with continuation of treatment. Nausea - prochlorperazine or metoclopramide. Switch from PI-based to INSTI- or NNRTI-based regimen.
Cholelithiasis	
Agent	ATV
ADR features	Abd pain; may cause cholecystitis, choledocholithiasis, pancreatitis, cholangitis
Monitoring	Consider RUQ US with abd pain (median onset 42 months)
Intervention	d/c ATV
Peripheral neuropathy	
Agent	ddI and d4T
ADR Features	Paresthesias and pain of lower extremities after weeks to months d4T also associated with rare cases of ascending neuromuscular weakness
Frequency	10-30% (or more) based on duration and dose
Monitor	Warn patient: Symptoms of decreased LE vibratory sensation and ankle jerk reflexes.
Intervention	D/C implicated agent. Possibly reversible if drug stopped early. Symptomatic treatment - pain meds, foot bridge, etc. Reversible if drug stopped early. Treat pain with gabapentin (most expensive), tricyclics, lamotrigine, oxycarbamazepine, tramadol, topiramate, and/or narcotics, topical lidocaine or capsaicin.
Rash	
Agent	NNRTIs (NVP, EFV, ETR, RPV), PI, (ATV, DRV/r, LPV/r, FPV, TPV/r,) InSTI, (RAL, EVG/c), MVC, ABC, and Ibalizumab (2 cases of severe rash reported)
ADR Features	Maculopapular ± pruritus -- Rare cases SJS, TEN
Frequency	NVP & EFV-15%, FPV-20%, ABC-5%, TPV/r-10-14%, ETR-9%, RPV-3%, DRV-7%
Monitor	Warn patient
Intervention	R/O, NNRTI-associated Stevens-Johnson syndrome or TEN and ABC hypersensitivity. Also R/O rash due to HIV-associated dermatologic complications and drug rashes due to other meds especially TMP-SMX, dapsone etc. Can often 'treat through' maculopapular rashes, but must D/C if progressive.

TABLE 11: Adverse Reactions of Antiretroviral Agents

Miscellaneous Reactions (cont.)	
Myopathy	
Agent	AZT>>RAL; DTG (Increased CK and myositis); BIC (increased CK)
ADR features	Increased CPK, muscle weakness and rhabdomyolysis
Monitor	Warn patient
Intervention	D/C AZT or RAL
Insulin resistance	
Agent	PIs (except ATV): IDV>LPV; AZT, d4T, ddI
ADR Features	FBS > 126 mg/dL ± symptoms of diabetes
Frequency	3-5%; higher frequency with family history of diabetes
Monitor	FBS at baseline, 3 mos, and then q3-6mos
Intervention	Switch to NNRTI- or InSTI-based ART regimen.Diet and exercise, metformin or rosiglitazone (no drug interactions with PIs) if indicated; may need insulin.
Hyperlipidemia / Cardiovascular disease	
Agent	Rank order to increase lipids: TPV/r>>LPV/r=FPV/r>IDV/r>SQV/r>EFV>DRV/r; ATV/r >ATV; dEVG/c; ABC, d4T, AZT; TAF> TDF. Minimal effect on Lipids: RAL, DTG, BIC, RPV, DOR Rank order to increase cardiovascular risk: ABC>ddI; FPV, IDV, LPV/r, DRV/r QTc prolongation: RPV (dose dependent)>EFV>SQV/r, LPV/r
ADR Features	Increased total and LDL cholesterol and triglycerides; Triglycerides. Begins within weeks.
Frequency	Variable
Monitor	Fasting lipid profile at baseline, 3-6 mos, and then annually.
Intervention	Based on National Cholesterol Education Program (Stone N. Circulation 2014; 129 Suppl 2: S1-45). See Page 31 Preferred statins: pitavastatin, atorvastatin, or rosuvastatin (with dose adjustment for co-administration with ARV if necessary.) Consider ART regimen change to InSTI based regimen (DTG, RAL, BIC) or RPV-based regimen.

Miscellaneous Reactions (cont.)	
Lipodystrophy: lipoatrophy and lipohypertrophy	
Agent	Lipoatrophy: d4T > AZT, ddI (when combined with EFV or PI/r) Lipodystrophy: EFV, PI/r, RAL + NRTIs
ADR Features	Lipoatrophy: thinning of buccal fat in face, extremities, and buttocks Lipohypertrophy: enlarged dorsocervical fat pad, abd visceral fat accumulation, and circumferential expansion of neck.
Frequency	Common with long-term use
Monitor	Self-image is most important
Intervention	Lipotrophy: avoid d4T or AZT (switch to TDF, TAF, or ABC). Changes are either slow to reverse or are irreversible. Injectable agents: poly-L-Iactic acid (Sculptra) can be considered.
Mental Status Changes Including Depression	
Agent	EFV > RPV>> DOR >ETR >DTG, RAL, EVG/c, BIC (unlikely w/ InSTI)
ADR Features	Spectrum includes confusion, impaired concentration, dizziness, abnormal dreams and depression. Possible increased risk of suicide or suicidal ideation Insomnia reported with DTG
Frequency	Up to 50% of EFV recipients; less frequent and severe with RPV (up to 9%)
Monitor	Warn patient of mental status changes including abnormal dreams; changes are noted immediately and usually improve with continued use over 2-4 weeks. Consider switch to PI- or ETR-based regimen. Caution patient regarding driving, operating heavy machinery and jobs requiring high level neurocognitive function. Symptoms reduced with initial EFV dosing on empty stomach since food increases absorption. Avoid EFV and RPV w/ history of uncontrolled depression and suicidality. Symptoms usually resolve with alternative regimen.
Bone Mineral Density (osteoporosis)[Brown TT et al. CID 2015]	
Agent	TDF+PI/r > TDF > PI/r >>> TAF , RAL , ABC
ADR Features	Decreased BMD, osteopenia, osteoporosis
Frequency	2%-6% reduction in BMD (varies w/ specific ART)
Monitor	Fracture risk assessment tool for all pts 40 yrs and older. DEXA scan for men (50 yrs and older), post-menopausal women, history of fragility fracture, chronic steroid (>3 months), and high risk of fall.
Interventions	Avoid TDF and/or PI/r in at-risk patients. Switch to ABC or TAF and RAL. Evaluate secondary causes of osteoporosis (e.g Vit D deficiency, hyperparathyroidism, subclinical hyperthyroidism, cushing, phos wasting)

TABLE 12: Antiretroviral Agents - "Black Box" Warnings

Agent	Reaction
Abacavir	• Fatal upon rechallenge in patients with hypersensitivity reactions: Do not restart if hypersensitivity reaction cannot be ruled out. (No reported cases with negative HLA B*5701 screening) • Lactic acidosis and steatosis*
Atazanavir**	None
Bictegravir/TAF/FTC	• HBV flare (HBsAg) when D/C TAF/FTC. May need to treat HBV.
Darunavir**	None
Delavirdine	None
Didanosine	• Fatal and nonfatal pancreatitis: Do not restart • Lactic acidosis with steatosis • Fatal lactic acidosis when combined with stavudine in pregnancy
Dolutegravir	None
Doravirine	None
Efavirenz	None
Elvitegravir	None
Emtricitabine	• Lactic acidosis with steatosis* • HBV flare (HBsAg) when ARV is stopped. May need to treat HBV. • Safety and efficacy for HBV treatment is not established.
Enfuvirtide	None
Indinavir**	None
Lamivudine	• Lactic acidosis with steatosis* • Patients with HIV infection should receive only dosage and formulations appropriate for treatment of HIV (300mg/d). • HBV flare (HBsAg) when ARV is stopped. May need to treat HBV.
Lopinavir**	None
Maraviroc	• Hepatotoxicity with systemic allergic response (rash, ↑IgE)
Nelfinavir	None
Nevirapine	• Hepatotoxicity including fulminant and cholestatic hepatitis & hepatic necrosis, especially in females with baseline CD4 count > 250 cells/mm³; monitor intensively in first 18 wks of therapy. • Severe, life-threatening skin reaction including toxic epidermal necrolysis (TEN), Stevens-Johnson syndrome, etc. • Do not restart if there is serious liver injury or serious drug reaction.
Raltegravir	• none
Rilpivirine	• none
Ritonavir	• Potentially serious drug interactions with nonsedating antihistamines, sedative hypnotics, antiarrhythmics, or ergot alkaloids (see Table 16)
Saquinavir**	None
Stavudine	• Lactic acidosis with steatosis • Fatal and non-fatal pancreatitis when used with ddI • Fatal lactic acidosis when combined with ddI in pregnancy

*FDA warning with NRTI class; however, unlikely to occur with ABC, FTC, 3TC, TDF, and TAF
**RTV contraindicated drug combinations applies to boosted PIs (PI/r or PI/cobi)

TABLE 12: Antiretroviral Agents - "Black Box" Warnings (cont.)

Agent	Reaction
Tenofovir* alafenamide*/ emtricitabine*	•Lactic acidosis with steatosis •Not approved for HBV infection (but active against HBV) •Potential hepatitis flare when TAF is stopped in patients with chronic hepatitis B. Initiate approved anti-HBV therapy if indicated.
Tenofovir DF*/ TAF*	• Lactic acidosis with steatosis* • Flare of HBV (HBsAg) when antiretroviral is stopped. May need to treat HBV. • Use TDF/FTC for PrEP only after confirming patient is HIV-negative
Tipranavir**	• Clinical reports of hepatitis and hepatic decompensation with death. Increased risk of hepatitis in patients with chronic hepatitis due to HBV or HCV. • Fatal and non-fatal intracranial bleed.
Zidovudine	• Hematologic toxicity: anemia & leukopenia • Prolonged use may cause myopathy • Lactic acidosis and steatosis

*FDA warning with NRTI class; however, unlikely to occur with ABC, FTC, 3TC, TDF, and TAF
**RTV contraindicated drug combinations applies to boosted PIs (PI/r or PI/cobi)

TABLE 13: Cardiovascular Health (Kohli P et al. J Am Heart Assoc 2014; 3:e001098)

Category		Intervention
A	Antiplatelet	ASA 81 mg/d if 10 yr clinical atherosclerotic cardiovascular disease risk > 10%
B	Blood pressure	Goal: <140-150/90
C	Cholesterol	See table 14
C	Cigarettes	Prevention
D	Diet	BMI goal 18.5-24.9 kg/m2; waist <40 (male) and <35 (female)
D	Diabetes	Goal: Hgb A1C <5.7%
E	Exercise	Goal: 3 to 4 forty minutes sessions/week
H	Heart failure	Prevention and/or treatment

TABLE 14: 2013 American College of Cardiology and American Heart Association (ACC/AHA) Guideline on the Treatment of Blood Cholesterol to Reduce Atherosclerotic Cardiovascular Risk in Adults
(Stone NJ et al. Circulation 2014; 129: S1-S45

Recommendations for statin therapy to prevent atherosclerotic cardiovascular disease are based on 4 "statin benefit groups" listed below

Patient Group	Intensity of Statin Rx	**Recommended Statin w/ ARVs
Clinical atherosclerotic cardiovascular disease (ASCVD): Hx of angina, MI, coronary revascularization, stroke, TIA, or peripheral arterial disease	Age <75: High-intensity statin; lowers LDL-C by $\geq$ 50%	BIC, DTG, RAL, DOR, RPV, NRTIs, MVC: atorvastain 80mg*; rosuvastatin 20 mg PI/r, COBI: Start with atorvastatin 10mg, then titrate to 40mg/d OR rosuvastatin 10mg/d, then titrate to 20mg/d
	Age >75: Moderate-intensity statin; lowers LDL-C by 30-50%	BIC, DTG, RAL, DOR, RPV NRTIs, MVC, PI/r, COBI: atorvastatin 10mg/d; rosuvastatin 10mg/d; pitavastatin 2-4mg/d
Adult (>21 yrs) with Primary elevations of LDL–C >190 mg/dL	High-intensity statin; lowers LDL-C by $\geq$ 50%	BIC, DTG, RAL, DOR, RPV, NRTIs, MVC: atorvastatin 80mg*; rosuvastatin 20 mg PI/r, COBI: Start with atorvastatin 10mg, then titrate to 40mg/d OR rosuvastatin 10mg/d, then titrate 20mg/d
DM (age 40 to 75) with LDL–C 70 to189 mg/dL and without clinical ASCVD	Moderate-intensity statin; lowers LDL-C by 30-50%	BIC, DTG, RAL, DOR, RPV NRTIs, MVC, PI/r, COBI: atorvastatin 10mg/d; rosuvastatin 10mg/d; pitavastatin 2-4mg/d
No clinical ASCVD or DM with LDL–C 70 to 189 mg/dL and estimated 10-year ***ASCVD risk >7.5%	Moderate-to-high intensity statin; LDL-C by 30 to $\geq$ 50%	BIC, DTG, RAL, DOR, RPV, NRTIs, MVC: atorvastatin 10-80mg/d; rosuvastatin 10-20 mg/d PI/r, COBI: Start with atorvastatin 10mg/d, then titrate up to 40mg/d OR rosuvastatin 10mg/d, then titrate up to 20mg/d

* Atorvastatin may be decreased to 40mg if pt unable to tolerate 80mg
** Statins dosing added by authors based on ARV drug-drug interactions
*** ASCVD risk calculator (http://tools.cardiosource.org/ASCVD-Risk-Estimator/)

TABLE 15: Drug Combinations That Should Not Be Used

	Not Recommended	ART Agent	Alternatives
Alpha adrenergic blocker	Alfuzosin; Silodosin	RTV, DLV*, all PIs*, COBI*	Low dose tamsulosin or doxazosin
Anti-angina	Ranolazine	All PIs*and COBI, DLV	None
Antiarrhythmic	Flecainide, propafenone	LPV/r, RTV, TPV/r, DRV/r, SQV/r, all PIs*, COBI*	If benefit outweighs risk, amiodarone (except with TPV/r) may be considered w/ TDM and ECG monitoring
	Dofetilide	BIC, DTG, all PIs*, COBI*	
	Amiodarone, quinidine, dronedarone	IDV, NFV, RTV, SQV/r, DRV/r, TPV/r, PIs*, COBI*	
Anti-convulsants	Carbamazepine, oxcarbazepine, phenobarbital, phenytoin	Unboosted PI*, BIC, DTG, DOR, ETR*, RPV*, EVG/c, DRV/c, ATV/c	Levetiracetam
Anti-gout	Allopurinol	ddI	Alternative NRTI
Antihistamine	Astemizole, terfenadine	All PIs, DLV, EFV, COBI*	Loratadine, cetirizine, fexofenadine, or desloratadine
Antimycobacterial	Rifampin	All PIs and NNRTIs are contraindicated (except EFV) BIC, COBI, EVG*, MVC†, TAF**	Use rifabutin with PIs§ or Use rifampin with EFV 600 mg qhs, RAL 800mg bid; DTG 50 mg bid
	Rifabutin	BIC, DLV, TAF**	Azithromycin
	Rifapentine	All PIs*, NVP*, DLV*, EFV*, ETR*, RPV*, COBI*, BIC, EVG*, TAF**, DOR*	Rifabutin (except TAF)
Antineoplastics	Irinotecan Enzalutamide and Mitotane	Irinotecan: ATV, IDV PIs, EVG, BIC, DTG, COBI, NNRTIs, EVG	None
Beta2-Agonist	Salmeterol	RTV, LPV/r, all PI/r*, COBI*	Formoterol
Ca++ channel blocker	Bepridil	RTV, TPV/r, SQV/r, DRV/r, all PIs*, EFV, COBI*	None
Ergot alkaloid	Ergotamine	All PIs, DLV*, EFV, COBI	Sumatriptan
GI	Cisapride	All PIs, DLV, EFV	Metoclopramide
	Proton pump inhibitor	ATV, NFV, RPV	H2 blocker 12hrs after ATV, NFV, RPV

(continued)

* Added by authors based on pharmacokinetic principles and/or high potential for toxicity
§ See Drug Table 16 (page 36) for rifabutin and antiretroviral dose adjustments
† IV Midazolam may be used with caution as a single dose given for a procedure (w/ LPV/r, ATV/r, TPV/r).
# MVC 600 mg bid can be considered (limited clinical data)
**Although not recommended by FDA, high tenofovir intracellular conc. observed (CROI 2018 abst 282B)

Class	Not Recommended	ART Agent	Alternatives
Hep C drugs	See Table 18 (page 49)		
Herbs	St. John's wort	All PIs, DLV, EFV*, DOR, ETR*, NVP*, RPV, COBI, BIC, DTG, TAF	Alternative antidepressants
Lipid lowering	Simvastatin, lovastatin	All PIs*, DLV, COBI	Pitavastatin, pravastatin, rosuvastatin
Neuroleptic	Pimozide	All PIs, DLV, EFV, COBI	None
Aldosterone antagonist	Eplerenone	All PIs, DLV, COBI	Spironolactone
Psychotropic	Oral midazolam†, triazolam	All PIs, DLV, EFV	Temazepam, oxazepam or lorazepam
	Alprazolam	DLV, IDV, all PIs*	
	Trazodone	SQV/r, all PIs*, COBI*	Consider aripiprazole at 25% of the dose with PI/r then titrate.
	Lurasidone	all RTV and COBI boosted PIs*, EVG/c	
Pulmonary HTN Agent	High-dose sildenafil	RTV, LPV/r, all PI/r*, COBI	Dose-adjusted bosentan or tadalafil
HCN channel blocker	Ivabradine	All PIs, DLV, COBI	No alternatives. Use alternative ARVs
Libido enhancement (premenopausal women)	Flibanserin	All PIs, DLV, COBI	No alternatives
Contraceptive	Drospirenone/ Ethinyl Estradiol	ATV/c and potentially other PI/c, PI/r, and EVG/c	Alternative OC (see page 45)
Steroid	Dexamethasone (multiple doses)	RPV, All PIs*, NNRTI*, EVG*, COBI*	Prednisone
	Inhaled and intranasal fluticasone	FPV/r, LPV/r, RTV, SQV/r, TPV/r*, ATV*, DRV/r*, all PIs*, COBI*	Beclomethasone

* Added by author based on pharmacokinetic principles and/or high potential for toxicity

TABLE 16: Drug Interactions: Drug Combinations w/ ARVs

Class	Agent	ART / Modification
Antifungal	Itraconazole	• All PIs and COBI may increase itra; monitor for toxicities • PI/r & PI/c: itraconazole dose > 200 mg/d requires TDM • MVC: decrease MVC dose to 150 mg bid • EVG, BIC, DOR, RPV* may increase (SD). DTG and RAL(SD) • EFV and NVP decreases itraconazole 35% and 61%, respectively; ETR may also decrease itraconazole. Use TDM.
	Isavuconazole	• LPV/r increases isavuconazole AUC 96%; LPV AUC decrease 27% (consider other PI). Other PIs and COBI may increase isavuconazole: monitor potential for toxicities and use TDM. • EFV, NVP, ETR may decrease isavuconazole conc. Use TDM • EVG, BIC, DOR, RPV* may increase (SD). DTG and RAL (SD) • MVC: no data. Consider dose reduction to MVC 150 mg BID if symptoms of orthostatic hypotension.
	Ketoconazole	• PI/r and PI/c: PIs and ketoconazole may increase. • LPV/r, TPV/r, FPV/r, DRV/r, IDV/r: ketoconazole ≤ 200 mg/d • FPV: ketoconazole ≤ 400 mg/d
		• MVC: decrease MVC dose to 150 mg bid • EVG, BIC, DTG, RAL. Use standard dose.
		• NVP: ketoconazole AUC decrease 72%. ETR may decrease ketoconazole • RPV* AUC ↑ 49%, ketoconazole AUC ↓ 24%. • DOR AUC increased 206%. Use standard dose.
	Voriconazole	• RTV ≥ 400 mg bid is contraindicated. With boosted PIs (RTV 100-200mg/d), vori AUC decrease by 39%. PI/r may be considered with voriconazole with TDM or use alternative. • With unboosted PIs, vori and PIs may increase. Use TDM. • COBI: voriconazole and COBI conc. may increase. Use TDM • EFV 300 mg qhs + voriconazole 400 q12h. Use TDM. • ETR AUC increased 36% and Vori AUC decrease 14%. Use TDM • EVG, BIC, DOR, RPV* may increase (SD); DTG and RAL (SD) • MVC 150 mg bid
	Fluconazole	• ETR AUC increase 86%; fluconazole – no change. SD • NVP AUC increase 110%; monitor for ADR • PI/r; EFV, RAL, MVC, DTG use standard dose • With TPV/r co-administration do not exceed fluconazole 200 mg/d • EVG, BIC, DOR, RPV* may increase (SD). DTG and RAL (SD)
	Posaconazole	• ATV conc. increase 2-3 fold. Posconazole may increase. Use TDM. • FPV and posa levels decreased. Avoid • COBI and RTV boosted PIs: Posa may increase. Use TDM • EFV decreases posa AUC 50%. Use TDM • ETR conc. may increase. Use TDM • DOR and RPV* conc. may increase. SD • EVG and BIC may increase (SD); RAL and DTG. Use SD. • MVC: reduce MVC dose to 150 mg BID
	Anidulafungin Caspofungin Micafungin AmphoB Lipid Ampho Flucytosine Pentamidine	• Limited data. Drug-drug interaction unlikely • No change in caspofungin level with NFV co-administration. • Caspofungin level may be decreased with NVP, EFV, ETR. Consider caspofungin 70mg/d. • Ampho B and Pentamidine: avoid TDF. Use TAF if CrCL >30 ml/min

*RPV associated with dose dependent QTc prolongation. Monitor QTc in patients at risk for QTc prolongation

Class	Agent	ART / Modification
Opiate	Buprenorphine	• EFV, ETR: decrease in buprenorphine conc.; no withdrawal symptoms observed. • ATV: increase buprenorphine, decrease ATV. Avoid • ATV/r & DRV/r: increase buprenorphine concentrations 66% & 46%, respectively. Monitor for sedation. • TPV/r: decrease TPV and buprenorphine active metabolite; LPV: no change. SD • NVP (and likely RPV), DOR, FPV/r, BIC, DTG, RAL: SD • COBI: Buprenorphine increase 35%. Monito • With PI/r, PI/c, EVG/c: titration with sublingual or buccal formulations preferred over implant.
	Fentanyl	• PI/r, COBI, DLV: may significantly increase fentanyl concentration. Avoid and use alternative.
	Methadone	• NVP and EFV: significantly decrease methadone by 50%; monitor for withdrawal Sx and increase methadone dose. • DOR and ETR: no interaction • RPV: R-methadone decreased 16% • IDV and ATV: no interaction • PI/r: TPV/r, LPV/r> FPV/r, SQV/r, ATV/r, DRV/r decrease methadone conc by 48% to 16%. Monitoring for withdrawal symptoms with TPV/r and LPV/r. • Methadone decreases buffered ddI levels; use ddI EC (no interaction) • AZT AUC increased 29-43%. Monitor for toxicity • BIC, DTG, EVG, RAL, unboosted ATV, COBI, MVC: SD
	Meperidine	• RTV: nor-meperidine increase 47%. Monitor
	Morphine, Hydromorphone	• RTV (at steady-state) may decrease morphine concentrations. Titrate to effect.
	Oxycodone	• LPV/r: oxycodone increase 2.6-fold. With PI/r and COBI use low dose and monitor for sedation.
	Tramadol	• PI/r, COBI: may increase tramadol conc. Monitor.
Benzodia-zepines	Midazolam Triazolam	• PI/r, COBI: Contraindicated with oral midazolam and triazolam. Use lorazepam, oxazepam, or temazepam. Use single dose IV midazolam w/ caution; consider propofol for procedural sedation. • ETR: midazolam AUC decreased 31%. NVP and EFV may decrease midazolam and triazolam. Titrate dose. • BIC, DTG, RAL, DOR, RPV, MVC, NRTIs: SD
	Diazepam Clonazepam Chlordiazepoxide Estazolam Flurazepam	• PI/r, COBI: Benzo may be increased. Consider lorazepam, oxazepam, or temazepam • EFV, NPV, ETR: may decrease benzo. Titrate to effect • BIC, DTG, RAL, DOR, RPV, MVC, NRTIs: SD •Lorazepam, temazepam, and oxazepam preferred with PIs, NNRTIs, and COBI.
Hypnotics	Eszopiclone, Zaleplon, Zolpidem; Suvorexant	• RTV: zolpidem increased 27%. Use low dose zolpidem with PI/r and COBI • PI/r and COBI: no data. Hypnotics may be increased. Consider temazepam or low dose zolpidem. • Suvorexant not recommended with PI and COBI.

Class	Agent	ART / Modification
Anti mycobacterial	Rifabutin**	• All boosted PIs: standard dose PI/r + RBT 150 mg qd or 300 mg 3x/wk (monitor RBT levels) • Note: recommended dose higher than FDA labeling because HIV-infected pts have lower RBT exposures. • Unboosted PI (ATV, FPV, IDV, NFV): RBT 150 mg/d or 300 mg 3x/wk (monitor RBT levels). Consider boosted PIs. • EFV 600 mg/d +RBT 450-600 mg/d or 600 mg 3x/wk • RPV: RBT 300 mg qd plus RPV 50 mg qd • DOR:RBT 300 mg qd plus DOR 100 mg q12h • ETR, NVP, RAL, DTG, MVC: RBT 300 mg qd; standard ARV dose. ETR+DRV/r is NOT recommended with RBT. • EVG/c: RBT metabolite increased 625%, EVG Cmin decreased 67%. Avoid • ATV/c, DRV/c: RBT 150 mg q48h. Monitor RBT levels • BIC: avoid RBT; TAF: avoid RBT
	Rifampin	• All PIs & NNRTIs: contraindicated except EFV (600 mg/d) using standard doses of rifampin • NVP, ETR, RPV, DOR: Contraindicated • BIC, EVG/c, ATV/c, DRV/c: Contraindicated • MVC: Consider MVC 600 mg bid or use rifabutin • RAL: Consider RAL to 800 mg bid or use rifabutin. • DTG: increase DTG to 50 m bid. Use only in pts with no INSTI mutations. • TAF: Avoid. tenofovir AUC decreased 55%, but high active intracellualr metabolite observed.
	Rifapentine	• May decrease PIs, NNRTIs (except EFV), BIC, DTG, EVG, TAF. Avoid • RAL plus weekly rifapentine: use RAL 400 mg bid. Avoid daily rifapentine dosing with RAL.
	Bedaquiline	• LPV/r: bedaquiline AUC increased 22% (single dose study) to 3-fold (PK modeling). Monitor QTc and LFTs • NVP: no change in bedaquiline concentrations. • EFV: may decrease bedaquiline concentrations. • COBI, PIs: May increase bedaquiline levels. Use only if benefit outweighs risk. Monitor QTc and LFTs
Erectile Dysfunction Agents***	Avanafil	• RTV increased avanafil AUC 13-fold. Avoid all boosted PIs, DLV, and COBI.
	Sildenafil	• COBI, PIs: ≤ 25 mg q48h and monitor • ETR: Sildenafil AUC decreased 57%. Titrate
	Vardenafil	• COBI, PIs: ≤ 2.5 mg q72h
	Tadalafil	• COBI, PIs: start with 5 mg; do not exceed 10 mg/72h

** For the treatment of TB, most experts recommend rifabutin 150 mg qd with PI/r. Use Rifabutin TDM.
*** Interaction unlikely with RPV, DOR, BIC, DTG, RAL, MVC. With ETR, NVP, EFV: ED agents level may decrease. Titrate to effect.

TABLE 16: Drug Interactions: Drug Combinations w/ARVs

(cont.)

Class	Agent	ART / Modification
Lipid lowering agent	Simvastatin Lovastatin	• EFV: simvastatin decrease 68%. With EFV, ETR, NVP: may require simvastatin and lovastatin dose increase. • All boosted PIs and COBI: up to 30-fold increase. Contraindicated. Use pitavastatin, atorvastatin • DOR, RPV, BIC, DTG, RAL, MVC, all NRTIs: SD
	Atorvastatin	• All PIs may substantially increase atorvastatin levels -- 8-fold with TPV/r (avoid) and LPV/r; 4-fold with DRV/r; 2.5-fold with FPV/r. Start with atorvastatin 10 mg then titrate. • ATV/c and DRV/c-ATO AUC increased 9.2- and 3.9-fold, respectively. Avoid ATV/c and do not exceed ATO 20 mg/d with DRV/c co-administration. • EFV, ETR, (and NVP): may reduce atorvastatin levels by ~1/3 • RPV: no interaction • DOR, RAL, DTG, MVC, all NRTIs: interaction unlikely
	Pitavastatin	• No dose change with PIs, NNRTIs, INSTIs, and NRTIs • ATV: pitavastation conc. increase 31%. Use SD • DRV/r, LPV/r: no clinically significant change.
	Pravastatin	• No dose change for most agents. • EFV: pravastatin decreased 44%; titrate dose. • DRV/r, pravastatin AUC increases in some patients 81%, but can be up to 5X in others • LPV/r: pravastatin AUC increase 33%; monitor. • MVC: No data; use standard doses • DTG, RAL, BIC: interaction unlikely • COBI: no data.
	Rosuvastatin	• Rosuvastatin AUC ↑ 108% (w/ LPV/r), ↑ 213% (w/ ATV/r), ↑ 26% (w/ TPV/r), ↑ 48% (w/ DRV/r). Dose: 5-10mg/day • FPV and SQV/r may increase rosuvastatin levels. • ATV/c: and DRV/c: Rosuvastatin AUC increase 3.4- and 1.9-fold,respectively. Max ROS dose 10mg/d with ATV/c and 20mg/d with DRV/c co-administration. • BIC, DTG, RAL, all NNRTIs, MVC: interaction unlikely
	Cholestyramine/ Colesevelam	• Binds to both basic and acidic drugs. No data with ARVs, but ARV absorption may be affected. Avoid co-administration.
	Fenofibrate Gemfibrozil	• ARV drug-drug interaction unlikely
	Niacin	• ARV drug-drug interaction unlikely
	Omega-3 acid ethyl esters	• ARV drug-drug interaction unlikely
	Ezetimibe	• No interaction with LPV/r. Interaction with other ARVs unlikely.

Class	Agent	ART / Modification
Antidepressants	SSRIs (Citalopram, Escitalopram, Fluvoxamine Fluoxetine Paroxetine Sertraline)	• EFV and DRV/r: sertraline decrease 39% and 49%, respectively. Titrate to effect. • DRV/r and FPV/r: Paroxetine decrease 39% and 55%, respectively. EFV and ETR: no interaction. • EVG/c: no change in sertraline conc. SD • RTV: no interaction with escitalopram • PI/r, PI/c: may increase fluvoxamine • With NNRTIs and PIs, titrate SSRI to effect. • RAL: no change in citalopram concentrations. SD • MVC, BIC, DTG, RAL, DOR, RPV: Interaction unlikely.
	SNRIs (Duloxetine, Milnacipran, Venlafaxine, Desvenlafaxine)	• Duloxetine may be increased with PI/r. At steady-state PI/r may decrease duloxetine • Venlafaxine and desvenlafaxine may be increased with PI/r. The active metabolite Desvenlafaxine and milnacipran may be increased with ATV/r, but decreased with PI/r and NFV. • ETR, EFV, NVP: may decrease desvenlafaxine. Titrate • MVC, BIC, DTG, RAL, DOR, RPV: Interaction unlikely.
	TCAs (Amitriptyline, Clomipramine Desipramine, Doxepin, Imipramine, Nortriptyline) TetraCAs (Maprotiline Mirtazapine)	• RTV: Avoid desipramine co-administration • RTV or COBI boosted PI may ↑ TCA concentrations. Use with close monitor for ADRs (QTc prolongation, sedation) • SSRIs are preferred over TCAs with PI/r co-administration. • PI/r and COBI: may increase mirtazapine levels. Use low dose and titrate to effect. • MVC, BIC, DTG, RAL, DOR, RPV: Interaction unlikely.
	Bupropion	• LPV/r: bupropion ↓46%; other PIs may decrease bupropiron • PI/c: usual dose likely. • EFV: bupropion ↓55%. NVP may ↓bupropion. titrate • MVC, BIC, DTG, RAL, DOR, RPV: Interaction unlikely.
	Trazodone, Nefazodone	• RTV (200 BID): trazodone increased 240%. Wth PI/r start with low dose and monitor for CNS ADR and cardiac arrhythmias. • SQV/r: contraindicated w/ trazodone • PI/r and COBI: nefazodone may be significantly increased. Use with caution (monitor LFTs). • EFV, NVP, ETR: may decrease trazodone and nefazodone. nefazodone may increase all NNRTIs. • MVC, BIC, DTG, RAL: Interaction unlikely.

Class	Agent	ART / Modification
Stimulants	Atomoxetine, Dextroamphetamine, Lisdexamfetamine, Methylphenidate,' Modafinil	• PI/r, COBI: may increase modafinil, D-amphetamine, atomoxetine. • Modafinil may decrease PIs, COBI, EVG, MVC, RPV levels • Methylphenidate: no data, interaction unlikely
GI agents	Antacid	• Avoid co-administration with ATV, RPV, NFV, TPV/r. • Give antacid 4 hrs after RPV, ATV, NFV, TPV/r • EVG, RAL, DTG: decreased by ~50-70%. Give EVG or DTG >2hrs before antacid • Avoid Al and Mg antacids with RAL • Although manufacturer recommends CaCO3 w/ RAL, RAL AUC decreased by 54%. Avoid • With Mg, Al, Ca: Give cations 2 hrs after BIC.
	H-2 Blocker	• ATV: Administer ATV 2h before or 10h after H2 blocker or use ATV/r 300/100 (in PI-naive patients); in treatment-experienced patients, boost with RTV and give H2 blocker (do not exceed equivalent of famotidine 20 mg) separately; consider alternative. ATV/r 400/100 if used with H2 blocker and TDF • RPV: H2 blocker 12 hrs before or 4 hrs after RPV • EVG/c, RAL, BIC, DTG, DOR, MVC: SD
	PPI	• Unboosted ATV, NFV, DLV, and RPV: avoid • ATV/r: avoid in PI-experienced pts. In PI-naive, avoid if possible. Do not exceed omeprazole 20 mg/d • RAL AUC increased 212%. Use standard dose • No significant interaction with BIC, DTG, EVG/c, LPV/r, FPV/r, EFV, NVP
	Sucralfate	Sucralfate may decrease absorption of DTG and other ARVs. Administer ARVs 2 hrs before or 6 hrs after sucralfate.
	5-HT3 agonist	• ARV interaction unlikely dolasetron, granisatron, and ondansetron: SD
	Low dose erythromycin	• EVG, COBI, PIs, NVP may be increased • COBI, PI/r, DLV may increase erythromycin. Monitor QTc • RPV may be increased. Monitor QTc
	Eluxadoline	• PI/r and COBI: may increase eluxadoline conc. Dose: eluxadoline 75mg bid
	Prochlorperazine Metoclopramide Dronabinol	• PI/r may increased dronabinol conc., but significant interactions unlikely. • Metoclopramide may be decreased with PI/r at steady-state. • Prochlorperazine: no data; use low dose with PI/r and titrate.

Class	Agent	ART / Modification
Anti-Diabetes agents	Glipizide Glyburide	• PI/r, DLV, and COBI: glipizide and glyburide may be increased.
	Nateglinide Repaglinide	• PI/r, DLV, and COBI may increase nateglinide and significantly increase repaglinide. A 19-fold increase in repaglinide observed with other CYP3A4 inhibitor (itraconazole). Nateglinide preferred • ETR, EFV, NVP: may decrease repaglinide and nateglinide. Titrate to effect
	Pioglitazone Rosiglitazone	• Pioglitazone may be increased with PI/r, DLV, COBI. • LPV/r, NFV, EFV levels were not significantly affected by rosiglitazone. Rosiglitazone preferred with PI/r.
	Canagliflozin Dapagliflozin Empagliflozin Ertugliflozin	• PI/r: may decrease canagliflozin. Dose may need to be increased with CRCL >60 ml/min. • ATV and IDV: may increase canagliflozin. • ARV drug-drug interactions unlikely with danagliflozin, empagliflozin, and ertugliflozin.
	Sitagliptin Saxagliptin Linagliptin	• PI/r, COBI, NRTI, NNRTI: drug-drug interaction unlikely with sitagliptin • PI/r and COBI: Saxagliptin level may be significantly increased with PI/r, COBI, do not exceed 2.5 mg/day • Linagliptin: PI/r and COBI may moderately increase linagliptin level • EFV, ETR, NVP may decrease linagliptin and saxagliptin
	Metformin	• DTG and BIC: metformin conc. increased 79% and 39%, respectively. Use with caution or avoid with renal insufficiency.
Antihistamine	Astemizole Terfenadine (off market)	• Contraindicated with PI/r, DLV, and COBI. • Cetirizine, desloratidine, fexofenadine, loratidine can be used with PI/r and COBI.
Potassium Lowering Agents	Sodium Polystyrene Sulfonate (Kayexalate), Patiromer (Veltassa)	ARVs concentrations may decrease. Separate ARV administration 3 hours before or after potassium lowering agents.
Antigout	Allopurinol	• Avoid ddI. • No ARV drug-drug interaction with other NRTIs
	Colchicine	• Avoid colchicine with PI/r and COBI with renal and hepatic impairment. • With co-administration: Administer colchicine 0.6 x 1, then 0.3 mg one hour later for gout flare. Co-administer only when PI/r is at steady-state (10-14 days). No data with PI/c or EVG/c use with caution at steady-state.

Class	Agent	ART / Modification
Anti-convulsant	Phenobarbital, Phenytoin, Carbamazepine, Eslicarbazepine, Oxcarbazepine	• Combinations of COBI boosted PIs with designated anticonvulsants should not be co-administered. • Carbamazepine: ↓IDV and potentially other PIs (except DRV and TPV) and NNRTIs (EFV AUC ↓ 36%) • Phenytoin: ↓NFV, ↓LPV, and potentially other PIs (except FPV/r) and NNRTIs. Phenytoin levels also↓ with NFV, FPV/r, and LPV/r. Monitor level. • PI/r should be avoided or use with caution. With co-administration monitor anticonvulsant and PI conc. or consider valproic acid or levetiracetam†. Avoid unboosted PIs and once-daily LPV/r • RPV and DOR is contraindicated; avoid or use EFV, NVP, ETR with close monitoring. • MVC: 600 mg bid • BIC: Avoid. • RAL: close monitoring with phenytoin & phenobarbital. Avoid RAL with carbamazepine. • DTG AUC decreased 49% w/ carbamazepine. Avoid • EVG AUC decreased 69% with carbamazepine. Avoid • TAF ↓ 55% w/ carbamazepine. Dose TAF 50mg/d. Avoid TAF with phenytoin, phenytoin, oxcarbazepine.
	Valproic acid	• LPV AUC ↑75%, TPV/r may ↓ valproic acid • EFV: no change
	Lamotrigine	• LPV/r: lamotrigine AUC decrease 50% • ATV/r: lamotrigine AUC decreased 32%; unboosted ATV: no change; PI/c: no data. monitor levels • BIC, DTG, RAL, DOR, RPV: SD likely
	Ethosuximide	• PI/r, DLV, COBI may increase ethosuximide level • NVP, EFV, ETR may decrease ethosuximide level • BIC, DTG, RAL, DOR, RPV: SD likely
	Zonisamide	• PI/r, DLV, COBI may increase zonisamide level • NVP, EFV, ETR may decrease zonisamide level
	Levitiracetam Topiramate	• ARV drug-drug interaction unlikely
Antibiotic	Clarithromycin	• DLV, DRV/r, LPV/r, RTV, SQV/r, TPV/r: decrease clarithromycin dose in renal failure (500mg/d w/CrCL 30-60; 250mg/d w/CrCL <30) or use azithromycin. • ATV increases clari level; decrease clari dose by 50% • MVC: 150 mg bid • ETR, EFV, NVP: may decrease clari levels; consider azithromycin; clari may increase RPV and DOR. • EVG/c: avoid with CrCL <50. Clarithromycin 500mg/d with CrCL 50-60 ml/min. • BIC, DTG, RAL: use SD
	Other Antibiotics	• PK Interaction with ARVs unlikely with aminoglycosides, beta-lactams, clindamycin, ethambutol, fluoroquinolones, sulfa, vancomycin • Isoniazid, linezolid, metronidazole: monitor for neuropathy with long-term co-administration with ddI or d4T.

Class	Agent	ART / Modification
Anti-parasitics	Artemether/ Lumefantrine	• DRV/r, LPV/r: ~18% decrease in artemeter and 3-5-fold increase in lumefantrine concentrations. Monitor for ARV efficacy and ADR (e.g QTc prolongation). • PI/c and EVG/c : may increase lumefantrine levels. • EFV: artemether active metabolite decrease 75% and lumefantrine decrease 56%. Consider alternative ARV. • ETR: artemether active metabolite decrease 15% nd lumefantrine decrease 13%. • NVP: Artemether active metabolite decrease 37% (no change in one other study). Lumafantrine AUC decreased 25% to 58% in 2 studies and increased 55.6% in another. Monitor closely for efficacy.
	Artesunate/ Mefloquine	• LPV/r: dihydroartemisinin AUC decrease 49%. Mefloquine AUC decrease 28%. Monitor for efficacy.
	Mefloquine	• RTV AUC decrease 31%. Monitor for boosted PI antiviral efficacy.
	Atovaquone/ proguanil	• EFV, LPV/r, ATV/r lower atovaquone AUC by 75%, 74%, 46% respectively. Consider alternative. • Proguanil concentrations decrease by 38-43%. • Consider alternative malaria prophylaxis
	Atovaquone	• ATV/r: no change in atovaquone concentrations. • EFV: atovaquone AUC decrease 44-47%.Use alternative
	Quinine	• RTV: quinine concentrations increased 4-fold • LPV/r: quinine AUC decrease by 50%. • PI/r, COBI: Monitor for therapeutic efficacy and toxicity (QTc prolongation and cinchonism)
	Tinidazole	• PI/r and COBI: may increase tinidazole level. Clinical significance unknown; use standard dose
	Albendazole, amodiaquine, dapsone, paromomycin, pyrimethamine	• ARV interaction unlikely; use standard dose
BPH agents	Alpha blocker: alfuzosin, doxazosin, silodosin tamsulosin, terazosin	• PI/r, COBI: alfuzosin and silodosin are contraindicated; doxazosin may significantly increase; terazosin may increase. Start with low dose then titrate • PI/r, COBI: tamsulosin may be increased. Start with low dose and warn patient of orthostatic hypotension. • BIC, DTG, RAL, NRTIs, MVC, DOR, RPV: interaction unlikely. Use SD • NVP, EFV, ETR: may decrease all alpha-blockers. Titrate to effect.
	5-alpha reductase inhibitor: Finasteride Dutasteride	• PI/r, COBI: finasteride and dutasteride levels may be increased. • ETR, NVP, EFV: finasteride and dutasteride levels may be decreased. • BIC, DTG, RAL, NRTIs, MVC, DOR RPV: interaction unlikely

Class	Agent	ART / Modification
Anti-neoplastics	Antimetabolite (capecitabine, floxuridine, methotrexate)	• AZT: additive bone marrow suppression • PI/r, NNRTI, COBI, InSTI, MVC: interaction unlikely. Use standard dose.
	Cisplatin, oxaliplatin, hydroxyurea, mitomycin	• Hydroxyurea: increased toxicity (pancreatitis, neuropathy, lactic acidosis) with ddI co-administration. • AZT: additive bone marrow suppression • PI/r, NNRTI, COBI, InSTI, MVC: interaction unlikely. Use standard dose.
	Mitotane; Enzalutamide	• DOR: DOR conc. may be decreased. Contraindicated. Mitotane and enzalutamide may also decrease the conc. of PIs, COBI, NNRTIs, BIC, EVG, DTG. Avoid • MVC: MVC conc. may decrease. Consider 600mg BID.
	Camptothecin (irinotecan and topotecan)	• IDV, ATV: avoid co-administration with irinotecan • Interaction with topotecan unlikely
	Alkylating agent (Busulfan, cyclophosphamide, dacarbazine, ifosfamide, lomustine, thiotepa) Anthracycline (daunorubicin, doxorubicin, idarubicin)	• IDV: cyclophosphamide clearance decreased by 50%. No change in IDV level. • PI/r, COBI: may increase alkylating agents levels. • EFV, NVP, ETR: may decrease alkylating agents levels • MVC, BIC, RAL, DTG, RPV, DOR: interaction unlikely • Good clinical outcome observed with standard dose CHOP+PI-based regimen. Modified CHOP (50% of cyclophosphamide and doxorubicin) also effective, but higher rate of relapse.
	Antineoplastics	• Antiandrogen (bicalutamide, flutamide, nilutamide) • Aromastase inhibitor (anastozole, exemestane, letrozole) • Bexarotene • Estrogen receptor antagonist (fulvestrant) • Ixabepilone • Mitoxantrone • Podophyllotoxin (Etoposide, Teniposide) • Estrogen Modulator (tamoxifen, toremifene) • Tyrosine Kinase Inhibitor (dasatinib, erlotinib, gefitinib, imatinib, lapatinib, sunitinib) • PI/r, COBI: may increase conc. of chemo agents listed above. Use with close monitoring • EFV, NVP, ETR: may decrease conc. of chemo agents listed above. Titrate dose based on clinical response. • DOR, RPV, BIC, DTG, RAL, MVC: interaction unlikely. Use usual dose.

Class	Agent	ART / Modification
Antineoplastics (cont)	Taxane (docetaxel, paclitaxel) Temsirolimus	• PI/r, COBI: may significantly increase taxane levels. Severe toxicity reported with LPV/r and DLV co-administration with paclitaxel. Significant (2-3 fold) increase in temsirolimus expected. • EFV, NVP, ETR: may decrease taxane levels • MVC, BIC, RAL, DTG, DOR, RPV: interaction unlikely
	Vinca Alkaloid (vinblastine, vincristine, vinorelbine)	• ddI, d4T: may increase the risk of peripheral neuropathy with long-term co-administration. • PI/r, COBI: may increase vinca alkaloid levels. • EFV, NVP, ETR: may decrease vinca alkaloid levels • MVC, BIC, RAL, DTG, DOR, RPV: interaction unlikely
Contraceptives	Oral Contraceptives: Ethinyl Estradiol (EE)/ Norethindrone (NE), Norgestimate, Etonogestrel Levonorgestrel, Drospirenone	• ATV/r: EE decreased. Norgestimate and Norethindrone increased. Use at least EE 35 mcg. • IDV & ATV: do not exceed 30 mg EE • ATV/c and DRV/c: drospirenone increased 2.3- and 1.6-fold, respectively; ATV/c contraindicated. Use DRV/c with caution. Monitor for hyperkalemia. • DRV/r, LPV/r, EFV, FPV+/- RTV, NFV, SQV/r, TPV/r, and RTV: EE and/or NE levels decreased. Use additional method of contraception. Avoid FPV w/ EE or NE. • EFV decreases levonorgestrel, etonogestrel, norelgestromin conc. by 58% to 83%. Use additional form of contraception. • DOR, ETR, RPV, NVP: use SD • EVG/c: Norgestimate conc. increased 2-fold. EE decreased 25%. Monitor for ADR. Drospirenone: monitor for hyperkalemia • BIC, DTG, RAL, MVC, NRTIs: use SD
	IM and Subdermal Implant: Depot Medroxyprogest erone (MPA); Etonogestrel implant; Levonorgestrel implant; Ethinyl estradiol/ norelgestromin (transdermal)	• LPV/r: MPA and Etonogestrel increased ~50%. Use SD • LPV/r: EE AUC decreased 45% and Norgestromin increased 83%. Use SD • PI/c and Other PI. No data. Use additional form of contraception. • EFV and NVP: use SD IM medroxyprogesterone. • EFV: Etonogestrel (implant) decreased by 63-82%. Use alternative form of contraception. NVP: no interaction • EFV: levonorgestrel decreased 47%. Use alternative form of contraception. No interaction with NVP. • DOR, ETR, RPV, NVP, MVC: use SD
Contraceptives	Vaginal Ring: Etonogestrel/ Ethinyl Estradiol	• ATV/r: EE AUC decreased 26% and Etonogestrel AUC increased 79%. Use SD • EFV: EE decreased 56% and Etonogestrel decreased 81%. Use alternative or additional form of contraction.

Class	Agent	ART / Modification
Ca++ channel blockers	Bepridil	• Contraindicated with all boosted PIs, COBI, and EFV*
	Diltiazem Amlodipine Verapamil and other Ca channel blockers	• ATV/r: diltiazem AUC increase 125% • IDV: amlopidine AUC increase 89.8%, diltiazem AUC ↑ 26.5% • With PI/r and COBI: start low dose Ca channel blocker and titrate. Decrease diltiazem dose by 50% and monitor EKG • EFV decrease diltiazem AUC 69%; titrate to effect with EFV, NVP, ETR. • BIC: diltiazem may increased BIC conc. • BIC, DTG, RAL, MVC, NRTIs: SD
Beta-blockers	Metoprolol Timolol Carvedilol Propranolol	• LPV/r, ATV/r: may prolong PR interval. Use with ECG monitoring in pts with known conduction abnormalities. • All PI/r and COBI: may increase beta-blocker concentration
	Atenolol Nadolol Bisoprolol Labetolol	• LPV/r, ATV/r: may prolong PR interval. Use with ECG monitoring in pts with known conduction abnormalities. • PI/r and COBI: Pharmacokinetic interaction unlikely.
	Sotalol	• PI/r and COBI: Pharmacokinetic interaction unlikely. • RPV: may prolong QTc. Use with close monitoring
ACE inhibitors	Captopril, Enalapril, Benazepril, Ramipril, Lisinopril	• PI/r, COBI: may increase captopril, enalapril, benazepril, ramipril. Use low dose and titrate to effect. Interaction unlikely with lisinopril.
ARBs	Losartan, Valsartan, Candesartan, Irbesartan.	• PI/r, COBI: may increase losartan. Consider candesartan, irbesartan.
Misc Cardiovascular	Clonidine, Hydralazine	• ARV Interaction unlikely with clonidine and hydralazine
	Ranolazine	• PI/r, COBI: contraindicated • NVP, ETR, EFV: may decrease ranolazine level
	Eplerenone, Ivabradine	• PI/r, COBI: may significantly increase eplerenone and ivabradine concentrations. Contraindicated.
	Nitrates	• PI/r, COBI: may increase isosorbide mononitrate/dinitrate
	Digoxin	• SQV/r and DRV/r: increases digoxin 49% and 36%, respectively. Other PI/r may increase digoxin level. Monitor diig conc. • COBI: no significant change in AUC, but Cmax increased 41%. Use standard dose

* Contraindicated with EFV, but clinical significance unknown

Class	Agent	ART / Modification
Pulmonary hypertension	Bosentan	• PI/r: significant increase bosertan levels; co-administer bosentan 62.5 mg qd or q48h only after PI/r has been given for at least 10 days. • COBI: same bosentan dosing recommendations as with PI/r coadministration, but no data. Co-administer with caution. • NVP, ETR, ERV: may decrease bosentan levels • RPV, MVC, BIC, DTG, RAL, all NRTIs: Significant interaction unlikely • ATV: avoid bosentan
	Tadalafil Sildenafil	• PI/r and COBI: avoid high dose sildenafil • PI/r and COBI: after >7 days on PI/r or COBI, tadalafil 20mg/d (max 40mg/day). No data with COBI; co-administer with caution. • NVP, ETR, EFV: may decrease tadalafil and sildenafil. titrate to effect. • RPV, RAL, BIC, DTG, MVC: interaction unlikely. Use standard dose
Glucocorticoid	Systemic steroid	• RTV: prednisone active metabolite increased 31%. • PI/r and COBI: may increase prednisone and prednisolone. Dose adjustment may be required. Triamcinolone acetonide and systemic budesonide, betamethasone, methylprednisolone should be avoided. • PIs, DOR, RPV, NNRTIs, EVG, BIC, DTG, COBI may be decreased by dexamethasone at steady-state. Use alternative corticosteroid with >10 days co-administration.
	Inhaled/ Intranasal steroid	• PI/r and COBI: significant increase in fluticasone serum concentrations resulting in Cushing's and adrenal insufficiency. Avoid • Budesonide and ciclesonide levels may be increased. Avoid • Mometasone: no data; low systemic exposure • Beclomethasone preferred with all ARVs.
Antimigraine Agents	Dihydroergotamine Ergoloid mesylates Ergotamine	• All PIs, COBI, EFV: Contraindicated • NPV, ETR: may decrease ergotamine concentrations • MVC, NRTIs, RPV, RAL, DTG: interaction unlikely
	Almotriptan Elitriptan Naratriptan	• All PIs, COBI: may significantly increase almotriptan, elitriptan, naratriptan levels. Consider rizatriptan, sumatriptan, zolmitriptan • NVP, ETR, EFV: may decrease almotriptan, elitriptan, naratriptan levels. • MVC, NRTIs, RPV, RAL, DTG: interaction unlikely
	Rizatriptan, Sumatriptan, Zolmitriptan	• Interaction unlikely with ARVs

Class	Agent	ART / Modification
Immuno-suppressants	Cyclosporine	• PI/r, COBI: may significantly increase cyclosporine levels** • Target trough 150-450 ng/mL. Higher rejection rate post-renal transplant. Consider using tacrolimus or sirolimus instead. • EFV, NPV, ETR: may decrease cyclosporine levels
	Everolimus	• PI/r, COBI: may significantly increase everolimus levels**
	Tacrolimus	• PI/r, COBI: may significantly increase tacrolimus levels** • EFV, NPV, ETR: may decrease tacrolimus levels • Target trough: 5-15 ng/mL (lower rates of rejection with target close to 15mcg/mL)
	Sirolimus	• PI/r, COBI: may significantly increase sirolimus levels** • EFV, NPV, ETR: may decrease sirolimus levels • Preferred in patients with calcineurin-associated toxicity. • Target trough: 3-12 ng/mL.
	Thalidomide	• Avoid long-term co-administration with ddI and d4T due to potential risk of irreversible peripheral neuropathy.
	Mycophenolate	• NFV AUC decreased 32%. Avoid • ATV, IDV: may increase mycophenolic acid • LPV/r, TPV/r: may decrease mycophenolic acid. • NVP clearance increased. Consider alternative NNRTI • Interaction unlikely with DTG, RAL, NRTI
Anti-arrhythmic	Disopyramide IV lidocaine Mexilitine Procainamide	• PI/r, COBI: do not co-administer. • ETR, EFV, NVP: may decrease anti-arrhythmic levels. • DTG and BIC may increase disopyramide conc. Monitor • BIC, RAL, DOR, MVC, NRTIs: interaction unlikely • RPV: monitor QTc closely with CYP3A4 inhibitor
	Flecainide Propafenone Dofetilide Amiodarone, Quinidine Dronedarone	• PI/r, COBI: do not co-administer. If no alternative, consider amiodarone with close monitoring. • ETR, EFV, NVP: may decrease anti-arrhythmic levels. • BIC, RAL, MVC, DOR, NRTIs: interaction unlikely • RPV: monitor QTc closely • BIC and DTG: contraindicated with dofetilide co-admin.
Androgen	Testosterone	PI/c: may decrease testosterone
THC	Dronabinol	PI/r and COBI: may increase Dronabinol
Multi-vitamin w/ minerals	Iron and Calcium Supplement	Give BIC, DTG, RAL, EVG > 2hrs before cation administration.

** TPV/r may increase cyclosporine, tacrolimus, sirolimus initially, but at steady-state levels may be decreased

Class	Agent	ART / Modification
Anticoagulant*	Clopidogrel	• ETR: ETR may decrease the efficacy of clopidogrel; avoid if possible. EFV may also decrease clopidogrel biotransformation into an active metabolite.
	Prasugrel	• PI/r and COBI: RTV decreased prasugrel active metabolite by 38%. Monitor closely for prasugrel efficacy.
	Ticagrelor	• PI/r and COBI:may significantly increase ticagrelor concentration. Avoid • ETR, EFV, NVP: may decrease ticagrelor conc. Avoid
	Warfarin	• Monitor INR closely if given with any PI or NNRTI (especially EFV or RTV) • PI/r and RTV may decrease INR at steady state • ETR may increase INR • RAL, DTG: interaction unlikely • COBI may increase or decrease INR. Monitor closely
	Dabigatran	• PI/r and COBI: avoid if CrCL <30ml/min. • With PI/r: Reduce dabigatran dose to 75 mg bid w/ CrCL 30-50ml/min • DRV/c: SD per FDA labeling, but use with caution in patients with CrCL <50ml/min • NNRTIs, INSTI, NRTIs, MVC: use SD
	Endoxaban	• All PIs: may significantly increase endoxaban conc.For non-valvular Afib, endoxaban 60mg/d (CrCL 50ml/min to <95ml/min). For DVT and PE, endoxaban 30mg/day (use with caution w/ CrCL <50ml/min) • ??DRV/c: SD per FDA labeling but use with caution with CrCL <50 ml/min • EFV, NVP, ETR: may decrease edoxaban levels. • DOR, RPV, INSTI, NRTIs, MVC: use SD
	Apixiban	• PIs, COBI: no data. May increase apixiban; avoid in patients who require low dose (2.5mg BID). In patients who require 5-10mg BID, use 50% of dose, but avoid if >80 y.o, Scr >1.5, <60kg. • ATV/c: avoid
	Rivaroxaban, Betrixaban, Vorapaxar	• PIs: no data. May increase rivaroxaban, betrixaban, and vorapaxar; avoid co-administration. • ETR, NVP, EFV: may decreased rivaroxaban, betrixaban, and vorapaxar. • ATV/c: avoid rivaroxaban. • DOR, RPV, MVC, DTG, BIC, RAL, NRTIs: interaction unlikely, use SD.
	Heparin&LMWH	• Interaction unlikely. Use standard dose

Class	Agent	ART / Modification
Antipsychotic	Fluphenazine, Haloperidol, Loxapine Perphenazine, Pimozide Thioridazine,	• PI/r, COBI: contraindicated with pimozide • PI/r, COBI: may increase typical antipsychotic conc. Start with low dose and monitor for ADR (QTc prolongation, anticholinergic, EPS) • RPV: with PI/r or COBI administration with typical antipsychotic, monitor for QTc prolongation. • ETR, EFV, NVP: may decrease pimozide • BIC DTG, RAL, DOR, MVC, NRTIs: Interaction unlikely
	Aripiprazole, Brexpiprazole, Cariprazine Clozapine, Lurasidone, Olanzapine, Paliperidone, Pimavanserin, Perphenazine, Quetiapine, Risperidone, Ziprasidone	• PI/r, COBI: may increase aripiprazole, brexiprazole, cariprazine, perphenazine, quetiapine, risperidone, thioridazine, ziprasidone. Use 25% dose of brexiprazole and aripiprazole, then titrate. With initiation of PI/r or COBI, use 50% dose of pimavanserin and cariprazine (see FDA labeling) . Initiate other atypical antipsychotics at the lowest possible dose, then titrate. Monitor QTc with ziprasidone co-administration. • PI/r, COBI: significant (>9-fold) increase in lurasidone; avoid. • PI/r: may decrease clozapine and olanzapine at steady-state. • PI/r, COBI, NNRTIs: Interaction with paliperidone unlikely • ETR, EFV, NVP: may decrease brexipiprazole, cariprazine, lurasidone, pimavanserin, quetiapine, aripiprazole, risperidone, ziprasidone. Avoid cariprazine. Titrate other atypical antipsychotic based on clinical response. Olanzapine may be decreased with EFV. • RPV: monitor QTc with ziprasidone when PI/r is co-administered • BIC, DTG, RAL, NRTIs, MVC, DOR: interaction unlikely

TABLE 17: Drug Interactions: HCV Antivirals w/ ARVs

	PI/r	NNRTIs	InSTI	NRTIs	MVC
Sofosbuvir	DRV/r: SD TPV/r: may decrease SOF; avoid	EFV: SD RPV, DOR: SD	BIC: SD RAL: SD	TDF*/FTC: SD	No data; SD likely
Ledipasvir (/SOF)	ATV/r, DRV/r, LPV/r: SD	EFV: Ledipasvir decreased 34%. Use SD RPV; DOR: SD ETR, NVP: Ledipasvir may be decreased	BIC: SD EVG/c: avoid when combined with TDF.	TDF: SD, but avoid with CrCL <60ml/min. Monitor for nephrotoxicity when combined with PI/r, PI/c TAF: use SD	No data: usual dose likely.
Simepravir (/SOF)	DRV: avoid; increased SIM PI/r and Cobi: avoid	EFV: avoid ETR, NVP: no data; avoid RPV; DOR: SD	RAL: SD DTG; BIC: SD EVG/c: avoid	TDF*, ABC, FTC, 3TC, T-20: SD	No interaction: SD
Dasabuvir, ombitasvir, paritaprevir, ritonavir	Avoid: DRV/r, LPV/r, TPV/r, COBI. ATV: 300mg/d (without RTV)	EFV: Contraindicated Avoid: RPV, NVP, ETR.DOR: SD	EVG/c: Avoid BIC: SD RAL: SD DTG: SD	TDF*, FTC, 3TC, T-20: SD	MVC no data; avoid or consider 150 mg bid
Daclastavir (/SOF)	Decrease daclastavir to 30 mg/day with ATV/r, ATV/c, IDV, NFV, SQV Daclatasvir 60mg/d with ATV, FPV, FPV/r, DRV/r, DRV/c, LPV/r. TPV/r: avoid	EFV, ETR, and NVP: increase daclastavir dose to 90mg/d RPV and DOR: daclastavir 60mg/d	DTG, RAL, BIC: daclastavir 60 mg/d EVG/c or EVG/r: decrease daclastavir dose to 30mg/d	Daclastavir 60mg/d	Daclastavir 60mg/d; MVC standard dose
Glecaprevir/ Pibrentasvir	Avoid PI/r and ATV	Avoid EFV and ETR. RPV, DOR: SD	EVG/c: SD monitor LFTs RAL, BIC: SD DTG: SD	TAF and TDF: SD; monitor GFR FTC and 3TC: SD	No data: standard dose likely.
Grazoprevir/ Elbasvir	ATV, DRV, LPV/r, SQV, TPV/r: increase grazoprevir/ elbasvir concentrations 2 to 8-fold and may increase risk of LFTs elevation. Avoid PI/r and COBI.	RPV: SD EFV: significant decrease in grazoprevir and elbasvir concentrations. Avoid EFV, ETR NVP. DOR: use SD	BIC: SD RAL: SD DTG: SD EVG/c: Avoid	ABC, FTC, 3TC, TDF, TAF, T-20: SD	No data: standard dose likely.
Velpatasvir** (/SOF)	TPV/r: avoid ATV/r, DRV/r: SD COBI: SD	EFV, ETR, NVP: avoid RPV, DOR: SD	BIC: SD DTG, RAL: SD EVG/c: SD	TDF: use with renal function monitoring. TAF may be considered	No data: standard dose likely.

SD standard dose. *TAF may be considered, but no data.
**With voxilaprevir co-formulation, avoid ATV/r, ATV/c, LPV/r. Monitor LFTs with EVG/c co-administration
If ribavirin added to regimen, ddI and d4T contraindicated. Avoid AZT (additive anemia).

TABLE 18: HCV Antivirals Drug Interactions

	Sofosbuvir	Ledipasvir	Simepravir	Dasabuvir Ombitasvir, Paritaprevir, RTV	Daclatasvir	Velpatasvir ****	Glecaprevir/ Pibrentasvir *****
Acid reducing agents	SD	May decrease ledipasvir. Separate antacid by 4h;. Famotidine 40mg bid or omeprazole 20mg/d (max dose)	SD	SD	SD	May decrease velpatasvir. Give velpatasvir 4h before antacid. Famotidine 40mg bid or omeprazole 20mg/d (max dose)	SD
CYP3A substrate w/ narrow therapeutic index (see page 32-33)	SD	SD	May increase intestinal CYP3A4 substrates (oral midazolam)	Same contraindication with drugs listed for RTV. See page 32-33.	SD	Atorvastatin and rosuvastatin may be increased. Rosuvastatin 10mg/d (max dose) or use pravastatin	All Statins may be increased. Use lowest dose with close monitoring. Do not exceed cyclosporine 100mg/day.
CYP3A4 inhibitors (azole antifungal, macrolides)	SD	SD	May significantly increase simepravir levels. Avoid	Paritaprevir, dasabuvir may be increased. Dose not established.	Decrease daclatasvir to 30 mg/day	SD	SD
Pgp and CYP3A4 inducers***	Avoid	Avoid	Avoid	Avoid	Avoid	Avoid	Avoid
Anti-convulsant**	Avoid	Avoid	Avoid	Avoid	Avoid	Avoid	Avoid carbamazepine
Ethinyl estradiol	SD	No interaction SD	No interaction SD	Contraindicated. Potential increased risk of ALT elevation.	SD	SD	Avoid. Potential increased risk of ALT elevation.
Amiodarone*	Avoid	Avoid	Avoid	May increase amiodarone levels. Use with close monitoring	Avoid	Avoid	No data

SD standard dose;
*bradycardia reported when sofosbuvir (in combination with ledipasvir, simepravir, or daclastavir) was given with amiodarone.
**carbamazepine, phenytoin, phenobarbital, oxcarbazepine
*** rifampin, St John's wort, rifampentine
****digoxin and topotecan levels may be increased. Monitor Digoxin levels. Avoid topotecan
*****digoxin AUC increased 48%; dabigatran AUC increased 138%. Use with monitoring & dose adjustment

TABLE 19: Drug Interactions: NRTIs

Drug	AZT	d4T	ddI**	TDF/TAF
Allopurinol	No known interaction	No known interaction	• ddI ↑113 to 312%. Avoid	No known interaction
Atovaquone	AZT AUC ↑31%. Monitor for BM suppression	No known interaction	No known interaction	No known interaction
Cidofovir, ganciclovir, valganciclovir	Ganciclovir + AZT increases marrow toxicity; monitor CBC	No interaction between d4T and ganciclovir	ddI and oral ganciclovir: ddI AUC↑111% (po) and 50-70% (IV); use with caution or avoid	TAF and TDF maybe ↑ May increase levels of co-administered tubular secretion substrate drugs • Monitor for toxicity
Methadone	AZT AUC ↑43%; no dose change; monitor CBC	d4T ↓27%; no dose change	ddI EC: no interaction	TDF: No change TAF: No data. Interaction unlikely
Ribavirin	Monitor for severe anemia; in vitro inhibition of AZT activation; not shown in vivo	In vitro antagonism but not clinically significant	Magnifies ddI toxicity; contraindicated	• Ribavirin unchanged; no data on TDF level TAF: no data
ddI	Limited clinical data	Increased toxicity: pancreatitis, peripheral neuropathy, lactic acidosis; avoid	--	ddI ↑44% • > 60 kg: 250 mg/d ddI EC • < 60 kg: 200 mg/d ddI EC • Avoid if possible TAF: no data, avoid
ATV	AZT AUC unchanged but C_{min} ↓29%; significance unknown	No interaction based on clinical data	Buffered ddI: take ATV w/ food 2h before or 1h after ddI or use ddI EC; separate dosing due to food restrictions	TDF: • ATV AUC ↓25% • TDF AUC ↑24% • Avoid concomitant use unless ATV/r TAF: TAF AUC ↑91%; TAF 25 mg/d with ATV
LPV/r	No PK data, but interaction unlikely	No data; interaction unlikely	Take ddI on empty stomach and LPV/r with food	TDF: • TDF AUC ↑32% • Use standard doses and monitor for TDF toxicity TAF: TAF AUC↑47%; LPV <-> Use standard dose
TPV/r	AZT ↓35%; clinical significance unknown	No interaction	Separate dose of ddI EC by ≥ 2h	TDF: tenofovir AUC ↓ 9-18% TAF: may ↓ TAF. Avoid.
DRV/r	Interaction unlikely	Interaction unlikely	Take DRV/r 2h before ddI	TDF: tenofovir AUC ↑22% TAF: no change standard dose • DRV no change

**ddI buffer-separate by 2 hours with drugs that require an acidic pH for absorption (e.g ATV, RPV)

TABLE 20: Dose Adjustments with PIs and NNRTIs Co-Administration

	EFV	NVP	ETR	RPV§	DOR*
ATV/r	ATV/r 400/100 (with food) + EFV SD (avoid in PI-experienced pts)	Avoid NVP increase, ATV decrease	ATV 14%. Avoid, but unclear clinical significance	RPV 25 qd ATV/r 300/100 qd	DOR 100 qd ATV/r 300/100 qd
ATV/c	ATV/c 400/150 (with food) + EFV SD (avoid in PI-experienced pts)	Avoid NVP may increase, ATV may decrease	Avoid ETR may increase, ATV may decrease	RPV 25 qd ATV/c 300/150 qd	DOR 100 qd ATV/c 300/150 qd
DRV/r	DRV/r 600/100 bid EFV 600 qhs (with DRV mutations); consider TDM	• DRV/r 600/100 bid + NVP 200 bid • NVP 27%	DRV/r 600/100 bid + ETR 200 bid	RPV AUC 130% DRV SD DRV/r 800/100 po qd + RPV 25 qd	DOR 100 qd DRV/r 800/100 po qd
DRV/c	Avoid DRV and COBI may decrease	Avoid NVP may increase, DRV and COBI may decrease	Avoid ETR may increase, DRV and COBI may decrease	RPV 25 qd DRV/c 800/150 qd	DOR 100 qd DRV/c 800/150 qd
FPV	• FPV/r 1400/300 qd + EFV SD • FPV/r 700 bid + RTV 100 bid + EFV 600 qhs	FPV/r 700/100 bid + NVP 200 bid NVP Cmin 22%	APV 69%. Beneficial interaction. Avoid, but unclear clinical significance	DRV/c 800/150 qd or FPV 1400/200 qd + RPV 25 qd	DOR 100 qd DRV/c 800/150 qd
IDV	• IDV 800 q12h + RTV 200 bid + EFV 600 qhs	• IDV 800 q12h + RTV 200 bid + NVP 200 bid	Avoid	IDV/r 800/100 bid + RPV 25 qd	DOR 100 qd IDV/r 800/100 bid
LPV/r	LPV/r 500/125† bid + EFV 600 mg qhs	LPV/r 500/125 bid + NVP SD	LPV/r 400/100 bid + ETR 200 bid	RPV AUC 52%, LPV 400/100 bid + RPV 25 qd	DOR 100 qd LPV 400/100 bid
NFV	NFV SD + EFV SD	NFV SD † NVP SD ‡	Avoid	SD	SD
SQV	SQV/r 1000/100 bid + EFV 600 mg qhs	SQV/r 1000/100 bid + NVP SD‡	SQV/r 1000/100 mg bid + ETR SD	SD	SD
TPV/r	TPV/r 500/200 bid + EFV 600 mg qhs	NVP no change SD	ETR 76%; Avoid	SD	SD

All doses in mg; SD = Standard dose; TDM = Therapeutic drug monitoring
* RTV (100mg bid) Increased DOR AUC by 254%. Use SD.
** Suboptimal PK. Boosting with RTV preferred
† LPV/r 600/150 mg bid preferred in treatment-experienced patients
‡ Limited clinical data, dose not established
§ RPV concentrations may be increased with PI/r or PI/cobi. Consider monitoring QTc in patients at risk for QTc prolongation

TABLE 21: Dose Adjustments with InSTI and NNRTIs or PI Co-Administration

	DTG	BIC	EVG	RAL
ATV/r ATV/c	DTG AUC 62% w/ ATV/r DTG 50 qd+ ATV/r 300/100 OR ATV 400 qd ATV/c: no data; SD	BIC AUC 310%; avoid but clinical significance unknown.	EVG Cmin 38% w/ ATV/r; EVG 85 +ATV/r 300/100 qd No data w/ ATV/; avoid	RAL AUC 41% w/ ATV/r; use SD No data w/ ATV/c; SD likely
DRV/r DRV/c	DTG AUC 22% w/ DRV/r DTG 50 qd + DRV/r SD DRV/c: no change; SD	BIC AUC 74% with DRV/c co-admin; SD	EVG 150 qd + DRV/r 600/100 bid OR EVG/c/TDF/FTC + DRV 800 mg qd	RAL 400 bid + DRV/r SD or DRV/c 800/150 qd
FPV+/- RTV	DTG Cmin 49% DTG 50 BID + FPV/r SD (use only if no InSTI resistance)	No data; BIC may	No interaction EVG 150 qd + FPV/r 700/100 bid	APV: no change RAL 400 bid+ FPV 700/100 bid
IDV	DTG may increase No data; SD	No data; BIC may significantly	No data; avoid	RAL may increase No data; SD
LPV/r	DTG: no change DTG 50 qd + LPV/r SD	No data; BIC may	EVG AUC 75% EVG 85 qd + LPV/r 400/100 bid	RAL 400 bid LPV/r 400/100 bid
NFV	No data; SD likely	No data; BIC may	No data; avoid	No data; SD likely
SQV/r	No data; SD likely	No data; BIC may	No data; dose not established	No data; SD likely
TPV/r	DTG AUC 59% DTG 50 BID + TPV/r SD (use only if no INSTI resistance)	No data; BIC may or . Avoid	EVG 150 qd + TPV/r 500/200 bid	RAL AUC 24% RAL 400 bid+ TPV/r 500/200 bid Avoid RAL QD
EFV	DTG AUC 57% DTG 50 bid + EFV 600 qhs (use only if no INSTI resistance)	No data; BIC may . Avoid	No data. Avoid	RAL AUC 36% EFV 600 qhs+ RAL 400 bid
ETR	With co-administration, must be given with boosted PI (DRV/r) DTG 50* qd + ETR 200 bid w/ PI/r.	No data; BIC may . Avoid	ETR 200 bid + EVG/ATV/r 85/300/100 qd EVG/LPV/r 85/400/100bid EVG/DRV/r 150/600/100 bid	ETR and RAL Cmin 17% and 34%, respectively. ETR 200 bid + RAL 400 bid Avoid RAL QD
NVP	DTG 19%. Use SD	No data; BIC may . Avoid	May EVG Avoid	No data. Usual dose likely
RPV	DTG 50 qd RPV 25 qd	No data. Usual dose likely.	RPV may increase SD; monitor QTc	No data. Usual dose likely
DOR	DTG 36%; SD	SD	DOR may ; SD	SD

*DTG 50 mg BID with DTG-associated (or suspected) resistant mutations.
All doses are in mg
SD: standard dose

TABLE 22: Pharmacokinetic Enhancement
Co-administration PI or InSTI with COBI or RTV

	COBI	RTV
ATV	ATV/c 300/150 mg qd (co-formulation)	ATV/r 300/100 mg qd ATV/r 400/100 mg qd (with EFV)
DRV	DRV/c 800/150 mg qd (co-formulation)	DRV/r 800/100 qd DRV/r 600/100 bid
FPV	No data	FPV/r 700/100 bid or FPV/r 1400/100 qd
IDV	No data	IDV/r 800/100 bid
LPV	No data	LPV/r 400/100 mg bid LPV/r 800/200 mg qd (co-formulation)
SQV	No data	SQV/r 1000/100 bid or SQV/RTV 400/400 mg bid
DTG	No data. Minimal DTG boosting expected	Minimal DTG boosting expected
EVG	EVG/COBI/TDF/FTC 150/150/300/200 (co-formulation) EVG/COBI/TDF/FTC may be co-administered with DRV 800 mg once-daily (use only as a simplification regimen in virologically suppressed patients).	EVG 85 mg qd+ATV/r300/100 mg qd EVG 85 mg qd+LPV/r 400/100 mg bid EVG 150 mg qd+DRV/r/600/100 mg bid EVG 150 mg qd+FPV/r700/100 mg bid EVG 150 mg qd+TPV/r500/200 mg bid
RAL	No boosting effect Use SD w/ COBI	No boosting effect Use SD w/ RTV
BIC	No data. Minimal BIC boosting expected; Use SD	No data. Minimal BIC boosting expected; Use SD

SD: standard dose

TABLE 23: MVC Dose Adjustments with InSTI and NNRTIs or PI Co-Administration

Maraviroc dosing when given in combination with PI, COBI, NRTIs, NNRTIs, InSTIs.

	EFV	NVP	ETR	RPV	DOR
BIC DTG RAL	MVC 600 mg bid	MVC 300 mg bid	MVC 600 mg bid	MVC 300 mg bid	MVC 300 mg bid
NRTIs (TDF, ABC, 3TC, FTC)	MVC 600 mg bid	MVC 300 mg bid	MVC 600 mg bid	MVC 300 mg bid	MVC 300 mg bid
PI/r* (except TPV/r) +/- NRTI	MVC 150 mg bid	MVC 150 mg bid	MVC 150 mg bid	MVC 150 mg bid	MVC 150 mg bid
TPV/r	MVC 600 mg bid	MVC 300 mg bid	MVC 600 mg bid	MVC 300 mg bid	MVC 300 mg bid
COBI* +/- NRTI	MVC 150 mg bid	MVC 150 mg bid	MVC 150 mg bid	MVC 150 mg bid	MVC 150 mg bid
CYP3A4 inhibitor* (e.g Telithromycin, Clarithromycin, Erythromycin, Itraconazole, Ketoconazole, Voriconazole, Delavirdine)	MVC 150 mg bid	MVC 150 mg bid	MVC 150 mg bid	MVC 150 mg bid	MVC 150 mg bid
CYP3A4 strong inducer (e.g Carbamazepine Phenytoin Phenobarbital)	MVC 600 mg bid	MVC 600 mg bid	MVC 600 mg bid	MVC 600 mg bid	MVC 600 mg bid
Rifampin Rifapentine	Avoid or consider MVC 600 mg bid	Avoid	Avoid	Avoid	Avoid
Rifabutin	MVC 600 mg bid+ EFV 600 mg qhs + RBT 450-600 mg qd	MVC 300 mg bid+ NVP 200 mg bid+RBT 300 mg qd.	MVC 600 mg bid + ETR 200 mg bid (without PIs)+ RBT 300mg qd.	MVC 300 mg bid + RPV 50 mg qd + RBT 300 mg qd	MVC 300 mg bid + DOR 100mg bid + RBT 300 mg qd.

* manufacturer recommends avoiding boosted PI with MVC with CrCL <30ml/min. Although NNRTIs are also not recommended with MVC in patients with CrCL <30ml/in, the clinical significance is unclear.

ANTIRETROVIRAL THERAPY
TABLE 24A: Indications for ART: DHHS (Oct 25 2018)

ART is recommended for ALL HIV-infected persons regardless of CD4 cell count to treat reduce morbidity/mortality of HIV infection and to prevent HIV transmission*

Strength of recommendation based on rating described in table 24B:
CD4 count <350/uL: AI; 350-500/uL: AI; CD4 > 500/uL: AI
AIDS-defining conditions, including HAD (HIV-associated dementia) AI
Acute opportunistic Infections*: AI
Pregnancy: AI
Chronic HBV co-infection: AII
HIV-associated nephropathy: AII
Rapidly declining CD4 count (eg >100 cell/mm^3 per year) AIII
Acute HIV: BII
HCV-coinfection BII
Higher viral load (>100,000 c/mL) BII

* Initiate ARVs within 2 weeks of new OI including lymphomas and HPV-associated cancer
An exception is cryptococcal meningitis in which delay initiation of ART until after 10 weeks of induction/consolidation antifungal to avoid the consequences of IRIS. Earlier ARTs start may be considered in pts with severe immunosuppression (CD4 <50).In TB treatment-naive patients, ART should be started within 2 weeks if baseline CD4 <50/uL and may be delayed to 2-4 weeks if higher CD4 count, but within 8 weeks of TB treatment (2018 DHHS OI Guidelines).
DHHS Same day ART initiation at time of diagnosis is being evaluated in clinical trials

TABLE 24B: Rating Scheme for Recommendation

Strength of Recommendation	Quality of Evidence for Recommendation
A: Strong recommendation for the statement	I: One or more randomized trials with clinical outcomes and/or validated laboratory endpoints
B: Moderate recommendation for the statement	II: One or more well-designed, non-randomized trials or observational cohort studies with long-term clinical outcomes
C: Optional recommendation for the statement	III: Expert opinion

TABLE 25: What to start: DHHS Guidelines (Oct 25, 2018)

Preferred Initial Regimen*	Caution
InSTI-based regimens BIC/TAF/FTC (AI) DTG/ABC/3TC (AI) DTG+[TDF/FTC(AI) or TAF/FTC(AI)*] RAL +[TDF/FTC(BI) or TAF/FTC(BII)]	Use BIC/T/FTC only if CrCL >30 ml/min Use ABC only if HLA B*5701 negative patients Use TAF only if CrCL $\geq$ 30 ml/min Use EVG/COBI/TDF/FTC only if CrCL $\geq$70 ml/min Use TDF only if CrCL $\geq$ 60 ml/min TAF has lower rates of nephrotoxicity and osteoporosis compared to TDF. Before DTG initation discuss risks of neural tube defects.Avoid DTG if pregnant and within 12 weeks of conception, planning to become pregnant, or childbearing potential without effective contraception

Initial Regimen in Certain Clinical Situation	Caution
PI-based regimens DRV/r(AI) or DRV/c(AI) + tenofovir/FTC [ATV/c or ATV/r] + tenofovir/FTC (BI) [DRV/c or DRV/r] + ABC/3TC (BII)	Use TDF only if CrCL $\geq$ 60 ml/min Use TAF only if CrCL $\geq$ 30 mL/min DRV is preferred over ATV generally Use ABC only if HLA B*5701 negative.
NNRTI-based regimens EFV/TDF/FTC (BI) EFV + TAF/FTC (BII) RPV/TAF/FTC (BI) RPV/TDF/FTC (BI) DOR/TDF/3TC(BI) or DOR+TAF/FTC(BIII)	Use RPV-based regimen only if VL <100,000 c/mL and CD4 >200/mm^3 Consider DOR-regimen if unable to take EFV or RPV based regimen
InSTI-based regimens RAL + ABC/3TC (CII) EVG/COBI/TAF/FTC (BI) EVG/COBI/TDF/FTC (BI)	RAL+ ABC/3TC regimen Only if VL <100,000 c/mL and HLA B*5701 negative.

Regimen when TAF, TDF, and ABC contraindicated	Caution
DTG plus 3TC (BI) DRV/r + RAL bid (CI) DRV/r once daily + 3TC (CI)	Use DRV+RAL only if pre-treatment VL <100,000 copies/mL and CD4 >200 mm^3

*Alphabetical order for combinations within major categories
3TC may be substituted for FTC or vice versa if non-fixed dose combination is desired. RAL can be given as 400mg BID or 1200mg once daily. TAF and TDF are two forms of tenofovir; TAF has lower rates of kidney and bone toxicity. Other NRTI-sparing regimens and 2 drug regimens are being studied.
T
Decision support is available at www.hivassist.com

TABLE 26: Advantages and Disadvantages of Initial ART Regimens: Adapted from DHHS Guidelines (October, 2018)

Drugs	Advantages	Disadvantages
Non-Nucleoside Reverse Transcriptase Inhibitors		
EFV	QD dosing; EFV/TDF/FTC coformulation; long term experience; potency with high viral load when combined with TDF/FTC.	Transmitted resistance more common than with other agents; CNS toxicity, including increased suicidality; dyslipidemia; drug interaction-CYP450; empty stomach preferred. QTc prolongation with high concentrations.
RPV	QD dosing; RPV/TDF/FTC (Complera) and RPV/TAF/FTC (Odefsey) co-formulation; small dissolvable pill. Better tolerated than EFV, including less CNS toxicity, lipid effects, and rash. RPV/TAF/FTC co-formulation may be used in patients with CrCL 30-69 mL/min.	Unlike EFV recommend only if VL <100,000 c/mL and CD4 >200/mm³; transmitted resistance higher compared to PI-based regimen (also more common compared with InSTI regimens); gastric acid and meal requirement; CYP450 inducer and inhibitor may decrease and increase RPV levels, respectively; RPV resistance with 138K mutation results in ETR cross-resistance; QTc prolongation with high concentrations.
Integrase Inhibitors (InSTI)		
DTG	QD dosing; superior to EFV and DRV/r due to better tolerability; higher barrier to resistance than EVG and RAL; Co-formulated DTG/ABC/3TC tablet; no food requirement; few drug-drug interactions. No transmitted resistance to date	4 case report of neural tube defects. Warning against usage in early pregnancy. Decreased absorption with Al, Ca, or Mg-containing antacid and vitamins; SCr elevation (no effect on true GFR); drug interaction with UDP-glucurosyltransferase (UGT) inducer (eg rifampin); coformulated only with ABC/3TC.
EVG/c	QD dosing; EVG/COBI/TDF/FTC (Stribild) and EVG/COBI/TAF/FTC (Genvoya) co-formulation. Lower LDL cholesterol elevation compared to ATV/r. EVG/COBI/TAF/FTC co-formulation may be used in patients with CrCL 30-69 mL/min.	Decreased absorption with Al, Ca, or Mg-containing antacid and vitamins; COBI causes SCr elevation (no effect on true GFR); Lower barrier to resistance than PI/r or DTG-based regimen; food requirement; drug interaction-metabolized via CYP3A4; ADR include H/A, transient diarrhea, nausea.
RAL	More post-marketing clinical experience than BIC, EVG/c and DTG; no food requirement; few drug-drug interactions Available as a once daily formulation for treatment naive-patients.	Decreased absorption with Al or Mg-antacid; BID dosing; low genetic barrier to resistance than PI/r and DTG-based regimen; ADR: CK elevation, myopathy, rhabdomyolysis; hypersensitivity reaction (including rare cases of TEN and SJS); drug interaction with UDP-glucurosyltransferase (UGT) inducer (eg rifampin). Higher pill burden than DTG and BIC

(continued)

TABLE 26: Advantages and Disadvantages of Initial ART Regimens: Adapted from DHHS Guidelines 2018 (cont.)

Drugs	Advantages	Disadvantages
BIC	Non-inferior to DTG/ABC/3TC and DTG+TAF/FTC Co-formulation with TAF/FTC No food restriction Well tolerated in clinical trials with less nausea compared to DTG/ABC/3TC	Less long term safety data compared to other integrase inhibitors. CYP3A4 inducer can significantly decrease BIC concentrations.
Protease Inhibitors		
ATV/r ATV/c	QD dosing; high resistance barrier when boosted with RTV or COBI; co-formulated with COBI No association with increased risk of CV events.	ADR: benign hyperbilirubinemia, cholethiasis, nephrotoxicity, nephrolithiasis, GI intolerance; drug interactions-CYP3A4 inhibitor; COBI boosting-avoid TDF with CrCL <70 ml/min.
DRV/r DRV/c	QD dosing; high resistance barrier; co-formulated with COBI DRV/c coformulated with TAF/FTC for single pill, once/daily regimen	ADR: Rash, GI intolerance; food requirement; drug interactions-CYP3A4 inhibitor; DRV/c: less clinical experience and unable to co-administer with NNRTIs; COBI boosting avoid TDF with CrCL < 70 ml/min. Association with increased risk of CV events in observational studies.
Dual-NRTI		
ABC/3TC	Co-formulated DTG/ABC/3TC tablet Good potency with VL >100,000 c/mL when given with DTG	Inferior virologic response w/ VL >100,0000 c/mL when combined with ATV/r or EFV; severe hypersensitivity reaction in HLA B*5701 positive patients; associated with increased risk of MI in some studies (debated issue despite extensive data)
TAF/FTC	Co-formulated EVG/COBI/TAF/FTC and RPV/TAF/FTC & DRV/c/TAF/FTC tablets. Lower rates of nephrotoxicity and BMD loss compared to TDF/FTC No dose adjustment for CrCL >30ml/min Active against HBV	Not yet recommended for PrEP Avoid TAF with CrCL < 30 ml/min No long-term data
TDF/FTC	Co-formulated EFV/TDF/FTC, EVG/COBI/TDF/FTC, RPV/TDF/FTC tablets; active against HBV; better virologic response at baseline VL > 100,000 c/mL than ABC/3TC when combined with EFV or ATV/r	Nephrotoxicity-proximal tubular dysfunction with acute and chronic renal insufficiency; nephrotoxicity risk may be increased with COBI or RTV-boosted PI administration. Avoid TDF with CrCL < 60 ml/min

TABLE 27: Factors affecting initial ART selection (DHHS guidelines October, 2018; decision support available at www.hivassist.com)

Factor	Recommendation	Concern or alternative
CD4 <200 cells/mm^3	• <u>Avoid</u> RPV-based regimen • <u>Avoid</u> DRV/r+RAL	Increased rate of virologic failure
VL >100,000 c/mL	• <u>Avoid</u> RPV-based regimen and DRV/r+RAL • <u>Avoid</u> ABC/3TC combined with ATV/r or EFV	Increased rate of virologic failure
HLA B*5701 positive	• <u>Avoid</u> ABC	High risk of severe ABC hypersensitivity reaction
No baseline resistance tests available or poor adherence	• <u>Avoid</u> NNRTI-based regimen and ABC-based regimen • <u>Use</u> DTG- (and likely BIC-) or DRV/r-+ tenofovir/FTC	Transmission of NNRTI resistant virus more likely than PI/r or InSTI
Convenience of one pill once daily	Fixed dose combination: • DTG/ABC/3TC (Triumeq) • EFV/TDF/FTC; EFV/TDF/3TC • EVG/COBI/TDF/FTC (Stribild) and EVG/COBI/TAF/FTC (Genvoya) RPV/TDF/FTC (Complera) and RPV/TAF/FTC (Odefsey) • DRV/c/TAF/FTC(Symtuza) • DOR/TDF/FTC (Delstrigo) • BIC/TAF/FTC (Biktarvy)	Use EVG/COBI/TAF/FTC and RPV/TAF/FTC only if CrCL >30 mL/min Use EVG/COBI/TDF/FTC only if CrCL >70 ml/min. Use RPV/TAF/FTC or RPV/TDF/FTC only if VL <100,000 c/mL an CD4 count > 200 cells/mm3
Food effects	<u>Must take with food:</u> • RPV-based regimen • ATV/r and ATV/c • DRV/r and DRV/c • EVG/COBI/TDF/FTC • EVG/COBI/TAF/FTC <u>Take on empty stomach:</u> EFV	Food improves absorption BIC, DTG, RAL, or DOR may be taken w or w/o food. Food increases EFV absorption and may increase CNS side effect (esp during the first 2 weeks). Can be taken with food if tolerated.
Renal disease	Avoid TDF* (esp. w/ boosted PI). Consider avoiding ATV If eGFR <70 ml/min: avoid EVG/COBI/TDF/FTC ATV/c + TDF/FTC DRV/c +TDF/FTC If eGFR < 60 ml/min: avoid ABC/3TC co-formulation If CrCL <30 ml/min, avoid TAF/FTC, EVG/COBI/TAF/FTC, and RPV/TAF/FTC	TAF or ABC-based regimen or DRV/r+RAL, DTG+3TC, or DRV/r+3TC can be considered instead of TDF. Use standard dose ABC and dose adjusted 3TC TAF may be used if CrCL >30 ml/min
Osteoporosis/ osteopenia	Avoid TDF	TDF may decrease bone mineral density with renal tubulopathy, urine phosphate wasting, and osteomalacia Use TAF or ABC

*dose adjusted TDF can be used in ESRD on HD

TABLE 27: Factors affecting initial ART selection (DHHS guidelines October, 2018) (cont.)

Factor	Recommendation	Comment
Psychiatric illness or HIV dementia or methadone maintenance	Avoid EFV Consider avoiding RPV Monitor patients on INSTI-based regimens with pre-existing psychiatric conditions. Consider DTG- or DRV-based regimen in pts w/ HIV dementia.	EFV may exacerbate psychiatric symptoms and confound assessment of HIV dementia improvement on ART. Methadone levels may significantly decrease with EFV co-administration. Methadone dose may need to be increased to prevent withdrawal symptoms
High cardiac risk	Consider avoiding ABC- and LPV/r-based regimen. If PI needed, use ATV. Consider BIC, DOR, DTG-, RAL-, or RPV-based regimens.	Increased cardiovascular risk seen in some in large cohort studies for the listed drugs. Among PIs, cohort stuides have shown some association w CV risk for DRV not seen for ATV. Consider avoiding RPV (and possibly EFV) in pts with prolonged QTc.
Hyperlipidemia	PI/r or PI/c (less with ATV and DRV) ABC, EFV, and EVG/c have been associated with increased serum lipids	DTG and RAL has minimal lipid effect TDF more favorable than ABC & TAF
Pregnancy/childbearing potential	Consider ATV/r, LPV/r, RAL PLUS TDF/FTC or ABC/3TC Avoid DTG-based regimen	Stay on current ARV regimen if VL <50 c/mL See pregnancy section (table 37)
HBV infection	<u>Use</u> TDF/FTC, TAF/FTC, (TDF or TAF) + 3TC. <u>If TDF or TAF cannot be used:</u> Entecavir + FTC or 3TC for HBV treatment (part of a fully suppressive ARV regimen)	TDF, FTC, and 3TC are active against HBV TAF (Vemlidy FDA approved) Use two active agents to prevent the rapid emergence of lamivudine resistant HBV. Severe HBV flare associated with TDF/FTC or TAF/FTC discontinuation with HBV-HIV co-infection
HCV infection	<u>Ledipasvir-Sofosbuvir:</u> use TDF with renal function monitoring when combined with PI/r or EFV or use TAF Daclastavir-Sofosbuvir: Daclastavir dose adjustment needed when combined with certain PIs and NNRTIs (see table 17)	See table 17 for all HCV drug-drug interactions Minimal drug ARV interactions with ledipasvir-sofosbuvir regimen.
TB co-infection	<u>With rifampin co-administration:</u> Use EFV 600 mg/d, RAL 800 mg BID, or DTG 50 mg BID (in pts without select INSTI mutations. see page 66); standard doses for DTG or RAL if rifabutin used. <u>If PI/r-based regimen needed:</u> use rifabutin (dose 150mg/d or 300mg 3x/week)	PI/r, PI/c, BIC, EVG, DOR, RPV, TAF co-administration with rifampin contraindicated Recent unpublished data (CROI 2018) suggests TAF is acceptable with rifamycins based on high tenofovir intracellular concentrations. Monitor rifamycin drug levels

TABLE 28: Methods to Achieve Readiness to Start ART and Maintain Adherence (DHHS 2018)

Patient-related methods

- Negotiate a plan or regimen that the patient understands and to which she/he commits
- Consider patient preferences: pill burden (frequency) and pill size, food effect, drug interactions
- Recruit family, friends, peer, and community support
- Use memory aids: timers, pagers, written schedule, pill boxes/medication organizers
- Plan ahead: keep extra meds in key locations, obtain refills
- Use missed doses as opportunities to prevent future misses
- Address financial issues: copays, insurance, etc.
- Active drug and alcohol use and mental illness predict poor adherence; race, sex, age, educational level, income, and past drug use do not

Provider- /Health team-related

- Educate patient re: goals of therapy, pills, food effects, and side effects
- Assess adherence potential before ART; monitor at each visit
- Ensure access at off-hours and weekends for questions or addressing problems
- Utilize full health care team; ensure med refills at pharmacy
- Consider impact of new diagnoses, intercurrent illness and events on adherence
- Provide training updates on adherence for all team members and utilize team to reinforce adherence
- Monitor adherence and intensify management in periods of low adherence
- Educate volunteers, patient-community representatives
- Treat mental illness (e.g., depression) and substance abuse

Regimen-related

- Avoid adverse drug interactions
- Simplify regimen re: dosing frequency, pill burden, and food requirements when feasible
- Inform patient about anticipated side effects
- Anticipate and treat side effects

Monitoring adherence

- Viral load – expect a decrease of 1-2 $\log_{10}$ c/mL by 4 weeks, VL < 400 c/mL by 8-16 weeks and then sustained levels < 20 c/mL: Documenting viral suppression is the most important metric for monitoring adherence since recommended regimens virtually always work (unless there is an unforeseen drug interaction or undetected baseline resistance). Note that viral suppression is the primary goal of treatment.
- Pill counts and pharmacy records are useful for documenting adherence

TABLE 29: Management of ART Treatment Failure

Virologic Failure

- Goal is to achieve suppression below limit of detection of available assays by 24 weeks. Expected response is a 0.75-1.0 $\log_{10}$ c/mL decline in VL by 1 week, 1.5-2.0 $\log_{10}$ by 4 weeks, VL <5,000 c/mL at 8-16 weeks and < 20 c/mL at 24-48 weeks.
- Virologic failure: Two consecutive HIV RNA levels > 200 c/mL after 24 weeks of ART
- Blip: After suppression, an isolated detectable HIV RNA level (200-400 c/mL) followed by return to suppression to <200 c/mL; not usually associated with subsequent failure
- Low level viremia: Confirmed detectable HIV RNA <200 copies/ml; significance unclear
- Causes: Poor adherence;Resistance (transmitted or acquired) which can reflect non-adherence; suboptimal pharmacokinetics from drug drug interactions, food requirements less common,
- Resistance test should be ordered (see below): Cost: genotype $300-400; Phenotype: $800-1200
- Boosted PIs (DRV/r; ATV/r) and all PIs have a high genetic barrier to resistance. Thus, most patients with viral failure on PI/r-based ART who fail will have sensitive strains of HIV unless the drug is continued with viral failure for prolonged periods. DTG also appears to have a higher barrier to resistance compared to RAL and EVG. Resistance to other antiretrovirals (esp NNRTIs, 3TC, FTC) occurs more rapidly when there is virologic failure.
- Resistance resources:Stanford University HIV database: http://hivdb.stanford.edu; IAS-USA: http://iasusa.org; HIV-ASSIST offers mutation evaluation and decision-support:www.hivassist.com
- Goal:Use at least two drugs in two classes that are active in vitro, and preferably three active agents.
- Considerations: 1)Never add a single agent to a failing regimen; 2) Do not stop ART since this leads to rapid VL increase and decrease in CD4 count, with potential for resistance, especially with NNRTI

Resistance Tests (see Table 31 Indications for Resistance Testing)

- Usually genotypic test, especially with early sequence failure.
- Testing should be done during therapy or within 4 wks of cessation of the failed regimen, if possible.
- Need for separate (or combined) InSTI genotype in patients failing InSTI-based regimens.
- A viral load of > 500-1,000 c/mL is usually required for the currently available resistance tests, but GenoSure Archive (proviral DNA) in patients with low or undetectable VL.
- Virologic failure of recommended first-line regimens are generally due to transmitted resistance or poor adherence.
- Phenotypic resistance assay can augment genotypic resistance tests in patients with multiple resistance mutations after multiple virologic failures. Especially useful in cases of complex PI resistance.
- For heavily treatment experienced, order Tropism assay to asses susceptibility to MVC

Using Resistance Test Results

- Interpretation of resistance tests results is complex and sometimes requires expert consultation.
- Resistance is cumulative: Interpretation should include history of prior ARV use and results of prior resistance tests. Past resistance mutations, even if not detected on the most recent test, remain relevant.
- Failure to detect resistance in the presence of failed treatment usually indicates non-adherence.
- Resistance tests are best for indicating drugs or drug classes that will not work rather than those that will work. Viral Tropism assay showing dual-mixed, or X4 virus suggests resistance to MVC

Immunologic Failure

- Failure to increase CD4 count 25-50/mm^3 during first year.
- Mean increase is about 100-150/mm^3 in first year with ART in treatment naive patients who achieve viral suppression; at 3-5 years the increase averages 20-50/mm^3/year.
- No data support switching ARVs when viral load is undetectable to improve CD4 response except for ADRs.
- Long term studies show that half of patients who start ART with a CD4 < 100/mm^3 never achieve a CD4 count > 500/mm^3. Attempts to improve CD4 response with methods other than viral suppression have been generally unsuccessful.

Clinical Failure

Occurrence or recurrence of HIV-related event reflecting HIV viremia $\geq$ 3 months after start of ART. Note: Must exclude immune reconstitution syndromes (IRIS).

TABLE 30: Management of Treatment Experienced Patients (DHHS Guidelines Oct 25, 2018; Viremia and Suppression)

Blips (<200 copies): Do not require change in ART; reassess Vl q3months

Low level viremia (>200 &<1000 copies): Persistent viremia in this range should be considered failure. Manage as with failure described below

Evaluation of failure: assess adherence, drug-drug interactions, drug food interactions, drug tolerance; HIV VL and CD4 count history; treatment history; prior and recent resistance test results

Resistance testing: Test during ART or within 4 weeks of stopping ART. Later testing still may be useful since resistance mutations may be detected.

ARV strategies with treatment failure:

1.Expert Advice: Should be sought; decision support available at www.HIVASSIST.com

2.New Regimen: Should include 2 active drugs (different drug classes) and preferably 3 total active agents

3.Virologic suppression not possible: Continue ART to maximize anti-HIV activity and minimize toxicity

4.Do not discontinue ART: Likely to result in rapid VL increase and decrease CD4

Additional Considerations: Active drugs are ARV's to which no resistance is seen on cumulative genotypes. Some mutations (M184V, K103N) are common after exposure to 3TC, FTC, or NNRTI's. If genotype is done off of ARV therapy, some resistance mutations may not be evident. In presence of some DRV resistance mutations, boosted DRV must be given twice daily to acheive higher drug concentrations; in presence of any INSTI mutations, DTG must be given twice daily

Optimizing ART in setting of Virologic Suppression: consider expert consultation

1. Fundamental principle is to maintain viral suppression
2. May be considered to: a)reduce pill burden or dosing frequency b)enhance tolerability by reducing short or long term toxicity c)mitigate drug drug interactions d)reduce costs
3. Review ARV history including toxicities, cumulative resistance tests, virologic responses
4. Monotherapy with INSTI or PI is NOT recommended
5. Within class switches may be possible provided there is no resistance to new ARV, and going to drug with higher/same barrier to resistance(e.g.,RAL or EVG to DTG; DTG to BIC; EFV to RPV; ritonovir boosted PI to cobicistat boosted PI)
6. Between Class switches can be considered provided no resistance (e.g., boosted PI to INSTI (DTG, EVG, or BIC); boosted PI to RPV; NNRTI to INSTI)
7. Two drug simplification: a)DTG/RPV shown effective in patients with suppression and no history of virologic failure. Consider when NRTI's not desirable or necessary. b)Boosted PI+3TC shown effective in patients wtih suppression and no prior risk of resistance
8. EVG/c/TAF/FTC+DRV as simplification in suppressed patients with prior failure

TABLE 31: Indications for Resistance Testing

Indicated
• Virologic failure with VL > 1,000 c/mL
• Virologic failure with VL > 500-1,000 c/mL, consider testing but may be unsuccessful
• Persons with suboptimal viral load reduction following ART initiation or switch
• Acute HIV infection; Baseline, (entry to care) prior to initial therapy

Not Indicated
• After discontinuation of antiretroviral therapy > 1 month duration. Positive results are helpful, but negative results do not exclude resistance mutations.
• With VL <1,000 c/mL, consider GenoSure Archive.

TABLE 32: Resistance Mutations 2017

(https://www.iasusa.org/sites/default/files/tam/24-4-132.pdf)

Drug	Codon Mutations
Nucleosides and Nucleotides - Reverse Transcriptase Mutations	
3TC	65R/E/N, 184VI
ABC	65R/E/N, 74V, 115F, 184V
AZT[1]	41L, 67N, 70R, 210W, 215Y/F, 219Q/E
d4T[1]	41L, 65R/E/N, 67N, 70R, 210W, 215Y/F, 219Q/E
ddI	65R/E/N, 74V
FTC	65R/E/N, 184V/I
TAF and TDF[1]	65R/E/N, 70E
Multi-nRTI resistance (TAMs)	41L, 67N, 70R, 210W, 215Y/F, 219Q/E
Multinucleoside Q151M plus	62V, 75I, 77L, 116Y, 151M
Multinucleoside 69 Insertion	41L, 62V, 69 insert, 70R, 210W, 215Y/F, 219Q/E
Non-Nucleoside Reverse Transcriptase Inhibitors	
EFV	100I, 101P, 103N/S, 106M, 108I, 181C/I, 188L, 190S/A, 225H, 230L
ETR[2]*	90I, 98G, 100I, 101E/H/P, 106I, 138A/G/K/Q, 179D/F/T, 181C/I/V, 190S/A, 230L
NVP	100I, 101P, 103N/S, 106A/M, 108I, 181C/I, 188C/L/H, 190A, 230L
RPV	100I, 101E/P, 138A/G/K/Q/R, 179L, 181C/I/V, 188L, 190A/S/E, 221Y, 227C, 230I/L
DOR	V106I, F227C

1 TAMs (induced by AZT or d4T) counteract selection of 65R
2 ETR: Most resistance requires 181C plus ≥ 3 baseline mutations to show reduced response.
* Tibotec Scoring System, weighted scoring system (based on DUET studies, HIV Med 2012; 13:427)
   • 3 points: 181I/V; • 2.5 points: 101P, 100I, 181C, 230L; • 1.5 points: 90I, 138A, 190S,
    179F; • 1 point: 179D, 179T, 101E, 101H, 98G, 190A:
     0-2 points: susceptible; 2.5-3.5 points: intermediate resistance;◦ 4+ points: high level resistance

Drug	Major**	Minor**
Protease Inhibitors - Protease Gene Mutations		
FPV/r	50V, 84V	10F/I/R/V, 32I, 46I/L, 47V, 54L/V/M, 73S, 76V, 82A/F/S/T, 90M
ATV[3]	50L, 84V, 88S	10I/F/V/C, 16E, 20R/M/I/T/V, 24I, 32I, 33I/F/V, 34Q, 36I/L/V, 46IL, 48V, 53LY, 54L/V/M/T/A, 60E, 62V, 64L/M/V, 71V/I/T/L, 73C/S/T/A, 82A/T/F/I, 85V, 90M, 93L/M
DRV[8]	47V, 50V, 54M/L, 76V, 84V	11I, 32I, 33F, 74P, 89V
IDV/r	46I/L, 82A/F/T, 84V	10I/R/V, 20M/R, 24I, 32I, 36I, 54V, 71V/T, 73S/A, 76V, 77I, 90M
LPV/r[4]	32I, 47V/A, 76V, 82A/F/T/S	10F/I/R/V, 20M/R, 24I, 33F, 46I/L, 50V, 53L, 54V/L/A/M/T/S, 63P, 71V/T, 73S, 84V, 90M
NFV	30N, 90M	10F/I, 36I, 46I/L, 71V/T, 77I, 82A/F/T/S, 84V, 88D/S
SQV/r	48V, 90M	10I/R/V, 24I, 54V/L, 62V, 71V/T, 73S, 77I, 82A/F/T/S, 84V
TPV/r[5]	47V, 58E, 74P, 82L/T, 83D, 84V	10V, 33F, 36I/L/V, 43T, 46L, 54A/M/V, 69K/R, 89IMV
Entry Inhibitors		
T-20	gp41 envelope -- 36D/S, 37V, 38A/M/E, 39R, 40H, 42T, 43D	
MVC[6]	X4 virus, dual or mixed tropic virus. Also mutations on HIV-1 gp120 V3 loop	

Integrase Inhibitors	Major	Minor
DTG[9]	148H/K/R, 263K	51Y, 66K, 92Q, 118R, 121Y, 138A/K, 140A/S, 151L, 153F/Y, 155, 230R
EVG[10]	66I/A/K, 92Q/G, 121Y, 147G, 148H/K/R, 155H	97A, 263K
RAL[7]	121Y, 143R/H/C, 148H/K/R, 155H	74M, 92Q, 97A, 138A/K, 140A/S, 263K
BIC[9]	148H/K/R, 263K	51Y, 66K, 92Q, 118R, 121Y, 138A/K, 140A/S, 151L, 153F/Y, 155, 230R

** Major mutations usually develop first and are usually associated with decreased drug binding; Minor mutations also contribute to drug resistance; may affect drug binding in vitro less than primary mutations. Use of Major and Minor designations for NRTIs and NNRTIs has been suspended.

3 ATV: ≥ 3 of the following mutations reduce viral response: 10FIV, 16E, 33FIV, 46IL, 60E, 84V, 85V. Another report implicates ≥ 3 of the following 10CV, 32I, 34Q, 46IL, 53L, 54AMV, 82FV, 84V.

4 LPV: ≥ 6 mutations required for resistance: 47A (and possibly 47V and 32I impart high level resistance.

5 TPV: ≥ 2 of the following mutations correlates with reduced response: 33G, 82IT, 84V, and 90M.

6 MVC: X4, mixed or dual tropic virus does not respond to MVC. Some mutations at codon 4, 11 and 19 of the V3 loop appear important but are not well defined and testing from commercial sources is not available. Emergence of X4 virus is more important.

7 RAL: Two major pathways: 148HKR or 155H with minor mutation. For 148HKR these are 74M plus 138A, 138K, or 140S. The most common and most potent cause of lost sensitivity is 148H and 140S. For 155H pathway the additional primary mutations with either 74M, 92Q, 97A plus 97A, 143H, 163K/R, 151I, or 232N. The sequential use of EVG and RAL (in either order) is not recommended due to potential for cross resistance. Lower barrier to resistance than BIC and DTG

8 With 0-2, 3, or ≥ 4 of 47V, 54M, 74P & 84V DRV mutations at baseline, the virologic response (< 500 c/mL at 24 weeks) was 50%, 22%, and 10% respectively.

9 DTG and BIC: Q148H and G140S w/ mutations 74I/M, 92Q,97A, 138A/K, 140A, 155H associated with DTG and BIC resistance. May retain activity against some RAL and EVG resistant virus. Additonal mutations listed based on reduced sensitivity similar to 155H.

10 EVG: 97A may occur as a polymorphism and does not significantly decrease sensitivity without other mutations. The sequential use of EVG and RAL (in either order) is not recommended due to potential for cross resistance. Lower barrier to resistance than BIC and DTG.

TABLE 33: Indications for ART: WHO Guidelines for Resource-limited Settings July 2018 Guidelines for managing advanced HIV disease and rapid initiation of ART.

When to start
All HIV-infected patients regardless of WHO clinical stage and CD4 count
HIGH PRIORITY: 1) WHO clinical stage 3 or 4 irrespective of CD4 count. 2) CD4 count ≤ 350 cells/mm^3 3) All patients with active TB regardless of CD4 count 4) HBV/HIV co-infection with severe chronic liver disease requiring HBV treatment 5) ART should be offered to partner in HIV serodiscordant couple to decrease transmission to HIV-negative partner 6) All pregnant and breastfeeding women

Clinical Stages	
Clinical Stage 1	Asymptomatic or PGL, and/or normal activity
Clinical Stage 2	Weight loss < 10%, minor mucocutaneous conditions, zoster < 5 years, recurrent URIs, and/or symptomatic plus normal activity
Clinical Stage 3	Weight loss > 10%, unexplained diarrhea > 1 mo, unexplained fever > 1 mo, thrush, oral hairy leukoplakia, pulmonary TB in past year, or severe bacterial infection, and/or bedridden < 50% of days in the past month
Clinical Stage 4	CDC-defined AIDS (page 11) and/or bedridden > 50% of days in the past month

TABLE 34: Starting Regimens for Antiretroviral Naive Patients: WHO Guidelines for Resource-limited Settings; July 2018

Patient Criteria	Regimen
ARV-naive	Preferred: TDF+3TC (or FTC) PLUS (EFV or DTG)* Alternative: AZT/3TC + EFV; AZT/3TC + NVP TDF/FTC + NVP; TDF + 3TC + NVP TDF/FTC + EFV 400mg*; TDF + 3TC + EFV 400mg* Not recommended: d4T-based regimens due to toxicities
TB co-infection	Preferred: TDF/3TC/EFV (with rifampin) Start ART as soon as possible (within 8 weeks of anti-TB treatment) Start ART immediately (within 2 weeks) w/anti-TB drugs if CD4 < 50

*EFV 400 mg can be considered if EFV 600 mg causes significant CNS side effects.
DTG was added as preferred first line in July 2018; caution if given in periconception period

TABLE 35: When to Change ART Regimens: WHO Guidelines for Resource-limited Settings July 2018

Failure	Definition
Clinical*	New or recurrent stage 4 condition (Table 33). Exceptions are lymph node or pleural TB, candida esophagitis, and recurrent bacterial pneumonia; must rule-out IRIS
CD4 count	Fall to baseline level; 50% fall from treatment peak; or levels persistently < 100 cells/mm^3
Virologic**	VL > 1,000 c/mL on 2 consecutive measurement and at least 6 mo after ART initiation. This level is associated with clinical progression and rapid CD4 decline

**Viral load is recommended as the preferred monitoring approach to diagnose and confirm ARV treatment failure (at 6 and 12 mo after ART initiation, and q12 mo after) If viral load is not routinely available, CD4 count and clinical monitoring should be used to diagnose treatment failure

*Clinical disease progression: events occurring > 6 mos after starting ARV because events in the first 6 mos often represent IRIS. New or recurrent events in the first 6 mos meriting change in therapy are AIDS-defining conditions (WHO clinical stage 4). Consider changing therapy for these WHO clinical stage 3 conditions: weight loss > 10%, unexplained diarrhea or fever > 1 mo, oral hairy leukoplakia, severe bacterial infection, or bedridden > 50% of days in past month

TABLE 35b: What ART Regimen to Change to: WHO Guidelines for Resource-limited Settings July 2018

Initial Regimens	Preferred Second-Line Regimens*	Alternative Second-Line Regimens*
[NVP or EFV or DTG] + 2 NRTIs	Heat stable [LPV/r or ATV/r] PLUS 2 NRTIs (see below for NRTIs)	2NRTI+DRV/r or RAL + LPV/r
• AZT (or d4T)+ 3TC†	TDF + (3TC or FTC)‡ + [ATV/r or LPV/r]	TDF + (3TC or FTC)‡ + DRV/r
• TDF + (3TC or FTC)†	AZT + (3TC or FTC)‡ + [ATV/r or LPV/r]	AZT + (3TC or FTC)‡ + DRV/r

† 3TC and FTC are considered interchangeable; they are structurally related and share pharmacological properties and resistance profiles.
‡ 3TC can be maintained in second line regimens to potentially reduce viral fitness, confer residual antiviral activity, and maintain pressure on the M184V mutation to improve viral sensitivity to AZT or TDF. AZT continuation may prevent or delay emergence of the K65R mutation, but continuation leads to TAMs and cross resistance to all NRTIs.

*With failure of second-line regimens, if available clinicians should include 2 new drugs with minimal risk of cross-resistance by using new drug classes (e.g integrase inhibitors), second-generation NNRTI (e.g ETR), and PIs (e.g DRV/r), entry inhibitors (e.g MVC)

TABLE 36. PREGNANCY AND HIV (DHHS Pregnancy Perinatal Guidelines Dec 7, 2018)

Hot Line: The National Perinatal HIV Hotline (1-888-448-8765) provides free consultative service for all aspects of perinatal HIV care.

HIV testing: All pregnant women should be tested (with 4th generation HIV test) at entry to care; repeat if symptoms of acute retroviral syndrome. Repeat testing in third trimester for women at high risk of HIV acquisition (e.g., IDU). Expeditied test during labor if status is unknown, with consideration of IV zidovudine if positive

Registry: All cases of ART exposure during pregnancy-report to Antiretroviral Pregnancy Registry (http://www.apregistry.com)

Goal: Goal of ART is to maximally reduce VL to provide optimal maternal therapy and prevent perinata transmission. All pregnant women with HIV infection should receive ART to prevent perinatal transmission regardless of baseline CD4 count or viral load.:

Preconception Safe sexual practice counseling; partner PrEP if not supppressed. EFV no longer prohibited. Risk of neural tube defects with DTG in early pregnancy; do not initiate DTG if considering pregnancy. Consider ATV/r, DRV/r, EFV, RPV with 2NRTI. Risk of transmission low if suppressed; condomless sex limited to 2-3 days before/after ovulation can reduce risk further.

Risk reduction counseling: Women with HIV infected partners should be alerted to the high risk of neonatal transmission during acute HIV. PrEP should be considered.

Antepartum: **Initiate/continue ART as soon as diagnosed during pregnancy**.

-Perform resistance testing. Treatment should not be delayed while awaiting results of resistance testing. Initial regimen can be modified once results are available.

-Drug selection-ART-naive

Use DHHS guidelines for drug selection with appropriate attention to baseline resistance test results, comorbidities, convenience, adverse reactions, drug interactions, experience with use in pregnancy and risk of teratogenicity.

Favored Regimens (see Table 37): NRTI backbone plus anchor (INSTI, PI)

-NRTI backbone: ABC/3TC or TDF/FTC (TAF has insufficient PK/safety data) PLUS

-Preferred anchor: PI/r (ATV/r or DRV/r; LPV/r as alternative) OR INSTI (RAL; DTG not recommended <14 weeks from LMP, but is a preferred INSTI after 1st trimester, BIC and EVG/c not recommended)

Alternative anchor: NNRTI(EFV and RPV). EFV alternative due to CNS side effects. Initial concerns for birth defects in primate studies, but now considered acceptable given extensive experience in pregnancy. RPV and EFV can be coformulated with TDF/FTC. Less experience with RPV in pregnancy. Lack of data for DOR

Drug selection-ART Experienced: Continue regimen (including EFV) if viral suppression achieved and regimen is tolerated, unless toxicity or PK concerns. If early LMP<14wks, use alternative to DTG. Avoid TAF,EVG/c, BIC, Cobi-ATV/DRV .

—If ART experienced, and not on ART, choose and initiate based on prior resistance testing, prior ARV use, concurrent medications, and recs on ART in pregnancy above. Consider expert consultation; decision support www.HIVASSIST.com

Monitoring: VL at initial visit; 2-4weeks after ART initiation; monthly until VL<50, and then q3 months. VL at 34-36 weeks gestation to inform decisions about delivery. CD4 initial; q3-6mo. U/S as soon as possible to determine gestational age. Amniocentesis: Should only be done with VL < 50 c/mL at time of the procedure.

<u>Intrapartum:</u> Continue antepartum ARTduring labor and before scheduled C-section
— IV AZT: If HIV VL >1000 c/ml or unknown, give IV AZT near delivery and schedule C-section. May be considered for VL 50-999. Not required if on ART and VL<50
— C-section: Pregnant women with VL>1000 c/ml should be offered C-section irrespective of antepartum ART. Not routinely recommended solely for prevention of transmission if VL <1000 in late pregnancy (vaginal delivery recommended). C-section has not been proven to reduce MTCT if a) Maternal VL <1,000 c/mL b) Membrane rupture over 4 hours c) Patient is in active labor
— Artificial rupture of membranes (ROM) performed in setting of ART with viral suppression is not associated with increased risk of MTCT
— If possible, avoid artificial ROM in setting of viremia.
— Generally avoid fetal scalp electrodes, or operative delivery with forceps/vacuum though data is from pre-ART era. In the ART era, recent data suggest operative delivery may be safe option when virally suppressed, but should be reserved for clear obstetric indications
— Oxytocin suggested when prolonged labor after rupture of membranes.
— Note that ritonovir usage inhibits cP450 and decreases elimination of fentanyl, but data suggests epidural anesthesia is safe regardless of ART regimen

<u>Postpartum:</u> Continue maternal ART;review need for modifications considering preferred regimens for non-pregnant adults

— Contraceptive counseling and plan before discharge.

— USPTF recommends screening all women for postpartum depression

— Breast-feeding: US guidance has recommended avoidance of breastfeeding because maternal ART reduces but does not eliminate breastmilk transmission, and there are safe infant feeding alternatives available in US.

<u>Newborn:</u> All perinatally exposed newborns should receive postpartum ARV to reduce perinatal transmission;Initiate ARV within 6-12 hours of delivery
ARV strategies in newborn includes the following based on risk assessment:

1. ARV prophylaxis: one or more ARV drugs in newborn Without confirmed HIV
   — if Low risk of acquisition(mothers received ART and virally suppressed near deliver; others considered higher risk): 4 weeks of ZDV prophylaxis
   — if Higher risk of transmission: ZDV for 6 weeks + 3 doses of NVP within 48 hrs, at 48hrs after first dose, and 96 hours after second dose; consider empiric ART

2. Empiric therapy: Administration of 3-drug combination to newborns intended as preliminary treatment of HIV: 3-drug regimen with ZDV, 3TC, and NVP. Indicated for newborns at high risk of acquisition (e.g., mother only intrapartum ARV, acute HIV during pregnancy, detectable Vl at delivery). Optimal duration is uknown.

3. HIV therapy: for neonates with confirmed HIV. See guidelines for use of ART in pediatrics.

Maternal HIV status unknown: Rapid HIV test of mother or infant and either ARV prophylaxis or empiric ART therapy.

National Perinatal Hotline (1-888-448-8765)

TABLE 37: Antiretroviral Drugs in Pregnancy (DHHS Pregnancy and Perinatal Guidelines 12/7/2018)

Advisory	Drugs
Nucleosides and Nucleotides	
Preferred	ABC/3TC; TDF/FTC** or TDF + 3TC
Alternative Regimen	AZT/3TC
Insufficient data to recommend	TAF/FTC
Not recommended	ddI; d4T; ddI/d4T (contraindicated); ABC/3TC/ZDV
Non-nucleoside RT Inhibitors	
Preferred	NNRTI-based regimens are no longer preferred.
Alternative Regimen	EFV* (monitor for CNS side effects) RPV* (avoid in VL >100K or CD4 <200 cells/mm3)
Not recommended or insufficient data	NVP (Avoid in women with baseline CD4 > 250 cells/mm³; monitor for HSR) ETR (not recommended in ARV-naive pts) DOR has no adequate human data to assess
Protease Inhibitors	
Preferred	ATV/r* 300/100 mg once-daily DRV/r* 600/100 mg bid (avoid once-daily dosing)
Alternatives	LPV/r* 400/100 mg twice daily. Increase to 600/150 mg or 500/125 mg bid in 2nd or 3rd trimester.
Insufficient data to recommend	FPV
Not recommended	NFV (low efficacy), TPV (not recommended in ARV-naive pts), IDV/r (nephrolithiasis), high dose RTV (high toxicity and low efficacy); SQV/r (Not recommended if QTc and/or PR prolongation) ATV/c and DRV/c not recommended.
Entry Inhibitors	
Insufficient data to recommend	MVC
Not recommended	ENF (not recommended in ART-naive pts)
Integrase Inhibitors	
Preferred	RAL 400mg BID*; DTG after 1st trimester
Avoid	DTG (4 cases of neural tube defects reported). Avoid in the first 12 weeks of pregnancy), sexually active and not on contraception, or planning to become pregnant.
Not recommened or insufficient data	EVG+COBI (low serum concentrations in the 2nd and 3rd trimester and is not recommended); BIC-no data. Chemically similar to DTG DTG/RPV combination not recommended

* Combine with preferred two-NRTI backbone; avoid RAL HD 1200mg once-daily
** Preferred NRTI in HBV co-infected patients

TABLE 38: Recommendations for Clinical Scenarios (DHHS Pregnancy Perinatal Guidelines 2018)

Clinical Setting	Recommendation	
Pregnancy potential plus indications for ART	Initiate ART per DHHS guidelines; counsel regarding DTG risks	
Receiving ART and virally suppressed becomes pregnant	1. Continue most ART if viral suppression achieved (see Table 39; insufficient data on BIC and DOR; switch DTG in 1st trimester; switch DRV/c, ATV/c, EVG/c; add additional agents if on only 2 drugs). 2. Labor: Continue ART and give IV AZT at delivery†if VL >1000 copies/mL. IV AZT not required if undetectable VL. 3. Schedule C-Section at 38 wks if VL > 1,000 c/mL near delivery 4. For infants: see Table 37 and below. If mothers did not receive antepartum ART or received only intrapartum ART or had incomplete viral suppression: expanded prophylaxis or empiric therapy with AZT,3TC,NVP (treatment dose).	
Treatment-naive and pregnant	1. Initiate preferred ART: ABC/3TC or TDF/FTC <u>PLUS</u> ATV/r, DRV/r, or RAL (Alternative TDF/FTC/EFV or TDF/FTC/RPV); DTG can be used after 1st trimester	
Treatment-naive, CD4 > 500/mm^3 and pregnant	1. Initiate ART (preferred regimen above) to prevent perinatal transmission 2. ART post-partum is currently recommended to all individuals to reduce risk of disease progression and prevent sexual transmission, irrespective of CD4	
Prior ART, now off treatment and pregnant	1. Initiate ART based on history and current and prior resistance test results, with considerations above	
Acute HIV in pregnancy	1. Risk of transmission to fetus is very high due to viral load often > 1 million/mL 2. Rapid testing (4th generation test) and institution of ART ASAP.	
Treatment-naive and presents in labor	**Options**	
	Mother	Infant
	AZT IV† during labor + AZT/3TC x7d po post-partum, then continue preferred ART combination (see table 37)	AZT§ x 6wks plus 3 doses of NVP* (at birth, 48hrs, and 96h) plus 3TC**x 6 weeks OR Empiric HIV treatment with treatment doses AZT, 3TC, NVP
Untreated HIV+ mother with newborn infant	Infant: AZT x 6 wks plus 3 doses of NVP* in the first week of life plus 3TC** x 6 wks for newborn infants Mother: Evaluate feasibility and initiate ART	

† AZT intrapartum: 2 mg/kg/h x 1h, then 1 mg/kg/h until delivery
§ AZT for infant > or = 35 weeks gestation: 4 mq/kg po 12h x 6 weeks
                       30-34 weeks gestation: 2mg/kg po 12h x 2 weeks, then 3mg/kg x 4 weeks
                       <30 weeks gestation: 2mg/kg po 12h x 4 weeks, then 3mg/kg x 2 weeks
* NVP 8 mg (birth weight 1.5-2kg) or 12 mg (birth weight >2kg) first dose at birth,second dose at 48 hours, and third dose 96 hours after second dose, then consider 6mg/kg q12h x 2-6 weeks (for >37 weeks gestation at birth)
** 3TC 2mg/kg twice daily x 2 weeks, then 4mg/kg twice daily x 4 weeks

TABLE 39: Antiretrovirals Data and Concerns for Pregnancy

Agent	Human Studies in Pregnancy	Concerns
Nucleoside and Nucleotide Reverse Transcriptase Inhibitors		
3TC	Well tolerated, Good pharmacokinetics with high placental transfer to fetus; not teratogenic	If mother's HBV co-infected, possible HBV flare with discontinuation.
ABC	Good pharmacokinetics at standard doses w/high placental transfer to fetus; not teratogenic	Must screen for HLA-B*5701
AZT	Good pharmacokinetics w/ high placental transfer to fetus. Extensive studies showing efficacy in reducing MTCT	Bone marrow suppression and poor GI tolerance
d4T	Good pharmacokinetics w/ high placental transfer to fetus; not teratogenic.	Lactic acidosis, especially when combined with ddI
ddI	Good pharmacokinetics with low to moderate placental transfer to fetus; increased risk of birth defects	Lactic acidosis rates increased, especially when combined with d4T
FTC	Slightly lower level in 3rd trimester; use standard dose; high placental transfer to fetus; not teratogenic.	If HBV co-infected, possible HBV flare with discontinuation.
TDF	Lower AUC in 3rd trimester, but trough adequate; high placental transfer to fetus; not teratogenic in human and animal studies. Preferred if HBV-co-infected	Primate study shows reduced fetal bone porosity, Human studies showed no effect on intrauterine growth. Conflicting data about potential effects on growth outcome later in pregnancy. If HBV co-infected, possible HBV flare with discontinuation. Monitor renal function. PROMISE showed higher preterm deliveries and infant deaths (0.6% vs. 4.4%) than with AZT-based ART, but not observed in other studies
TAF	No PK or placental transfer data. Not teratogenic in animal studies	Insufficient data to recommend.
Non- Nucleoside Reverse Transcriptase Inhibitors		
EFV	Neural tube defects in primates study with exposure in the first 8 weeks, but human data does not suggest an increase in fetal risk (with > 2000 births). AUC decreased during 3rd trimester, but trough adequate in nearly all patients w/ moderate placental transfer to fetus.	An alternative ART due to increased risk of CNS ADR FDA pregnancy category D, but if VL <50 c/mL switching off EFV not recommended due to risk of loss of viral control and increased risk of perinatal transmission.
NVP	Good pharmacokinetics with high placental transfer to the fetus, safety and efficacy of single perinatal dose to prevent transmission shown in many trials. Not teratogenic	No longer recommended as an alternative ART in pregnancy. Concern is HSR/rash treatment naive patients with baseline CD4 count > 250 cells/mm^3
RPV	Concentrations decreased 20-30% compared to post-partum with high PK variability. Moderate to high placental transfer to fetus	Insufficient data to recommend routine use, but can be considered as an alternative NNRTI.
ETR	Concentrations increased by 20-60% in pregnancy. Not teratogenic in animal studies. Variable placental transfer (19% to 325% maternal serum concentration).	Not recommended in treatment-naive patients
DOR	With over 8X human exposure, not teratogenic in animal stuides.	Insufficient data to recommend.
Entry Inhibitor		
ENF	No PK data. Low placental transfer to fetus	Insufficient data to recommend routine use
MVC	MVC trough adequate in pregnancy. Low placental transfer to fetus. Not teratogenic in animal studies, but inadequate human data.	Insufficient data to recommend routine use

TABLE 39: Antiretrovirals Data and Concerns for Pregnancy
(cont.)

Agent	Human Studies in Pregnancy	Concerns
Protease Inhibitors		
PI Class	Diabetes, GI intolerance	Risk of diabetes and ketoacidosis; unclear if rate is increased in pregnancy
ATV	2/3 PK studies showed decreased concentration in the third trimester w/ low placental transfer to fetus. Not teratogenic Use ATV/r 400/100 with TDF or H2 blocker coadministration in ARV-experienced patient; some experts recommend ATV/r 400/100 in all women in the 2nd and 3rd trimester.	Hyperbilirubinemia. Non-pathologic elevations of neonatal hyperbilirubinemia in some, but not observed in all clinical trials. One of the preferred PI in combination with TDF/FTC or ABC/3TC in pregnancy No data with ATV/c.
DRV/r	Decreased exposure in pregnancy w/ low placental transfer to fetus. Not teratogenic in animal studies and no evidence of human teratogenicity. Use DRV/r 600/100 bid	One of the preferred PI when used in combination with TDF/FTC or ABC/3TC in pregnancy. No data with DRV/c.
FPV	AUC decreased 36% in 3rd trimester. Avoid unboosted FPV. Low placental transfer to fetus. Use FPV/r 700/100 bid	Safety in pregnancy data are insufficient to recommend use during pregnancy. With FPV/r, trough adequate in PI-naive patients
IDV	AUC decreased 50-80% in pregnancy w/ minimal placental transfer to fetus. Not teratogenic	Concern for hyperbilirubinemia, but low placental transfer to fetus mitigates this concern. Not recommended in pregnancy.
LPV/r	Decreased concentrations in 2nd and 3rd trimester w/ low placental transfer to fetus. Increase dose to LPV/r 600/150 mg bid in 2nd and 3rd trimester.	Once-daily dosing not recommended in pregnancy. Avoid oral solution in pregnancy due to alcohol and propylene glycol content. LPV/r can be used as an alternative PI/r.
NFV	PACTG 353 showed doses of 1250 mg bid achieved therapeutic levels (but not 750 mg tid). Minimal to low placental transfer to fetus. Not teratogenic.	Avoid use due to lower potency compared to LPV/r
SQV	Studies with unboosted Fortovase showed reduced levels in pregnancy; data for Invirase are limited. Low placental transfer to fetus. Not teratogenic in animal studies, but limited human data. Use SQV/r 1000/100 bid	Monitor PR and QTc interval. SQV/r is no longer recommended as an alternative PI/r.
RTV	Lower concentrations in pregnancy, but no dose adjustment needed. Not teratogenic. Low placental transfer to fetus.	Avoid oral solution in pregnancy due to alcohol content.
TPV	Limited PK data. Not teratogenic in animal studies, but limited human data.	Hepatitis; Avoid
Integrase Inhibitor		
DTG	Limited PK data. Not teratogenic in animal studies, but 4 cases of neural tube defects reported.	Test for pregnancy before initiating DTG-based regiment. Avoid in the first 12 weeks of pregnancy
EVG	Low conc. in 2nd and 3rd trimester. Not teratogenic in animal studies, but limited human data. Unknown placental transfer	Insufficient data to recommend routine use
RAL	Limited PK data suggest no dosage change in pregnancy. Not teratogenic in rabbit studies, but limited human data limited to fewer than 300 first-trimester exposure. High placental transfer	Preferred InSTI during pregnancy when combined with TDF/FTC or ABC/3TC. Reports of LFTs elevation late in pregnancy.
BIC	Insufficient Data	

TABLE 40: Mode of Delivery

Clinical Setting	Recommendation
HIV infected presents at > 36 weeks, on no ART, labs pending	1. Start ART per Table 38 for mother 2. Recommend C-section at 38 weeks 3. IV AZT to mother, then continue ART 4. Use prophylactic antibacterials 5. ART should be continued post-partum 6. Consider empiric HIV therapy (3 drug) for newborn
HIV treated, pregnant and VL > 1000 c/mL at 36 weeks	1. Continue ART if VL decreasing or change if poor virologic response 2. Schedule C-section if VL likely to be > 1000 c/mL at 38 weeks 3. Continue ARV through surgical period 4. Prophylactic antibacterials for the C-section 5. Continue ART 6. Consider prophylaxis (AZT 6wks+NVP/3TC, see above) OR empiric HIV therapy (3 drug combination ART)
Mother receiving ART with virologic control (VL <1000 c/ml	Risk of perinatal transmission is < 2%; C-section is not routinely recommended AZT for 4 weeks to newborn.
Mother has scheduled C-section but presents in labor	1. Give IV AZT to mother 2. Risk and benefit of C-section should be evaluated on a cases by case basis 3. Give post-partum AZT to infant

TABLE 41: Drugs to Avoid During Pregnancy

Agent	Class*	Recommendation
ACE Inhibitors and ARBs	D	Use alternative antihypertensive (methyldopa)
Warfarin	X	Consider heparin or LMW heparin
Anticonvulsants: carbamazepine, valproic acid, phenytoin, and phenobarbital	D	Can be continued if indicated. Consider alternate anticonvulsants.
HMG-CoA reductase inhibitor	D	Consider alternative (eg fibrinic acid, niacin)
Paroxetine	D	Consider alternative antidepressant
Miscellaneous: ergotamine, thalidomide, raloxifene, misoprostol, retinoids, and benzodiazepines	X	Contraindicated
ribavirin	X	Contraindicated

* FDA pregnancy category:
  A   controlled studies show no risk
  B   no evidence of risk in humans
  C   risk not ruled out
  D   positive evidence of risk
  X   contraindicated in pregnancy

TABLE 42: Drugs for Opportunistic Infections in Pregnancy

(DHHS Updated Prevention and Treatment of Opportunistic Infections, MMWR 2009;58:RR11)

Agent	Class*	Recommendation
Acyclovir	B	Treatment reserved for severe herpes or varicella; well-tolerated and no consequences with > 700 mg exposure
Albendazole	C	Teratogenic in rodents; reserve for severe microsporidiosis in 2nd and 3rd trimester
Amoxicillin	B	Standard indications
Amphotericin	B	Standard indications
Atovaquone	C	Standard indications; limited experience
Azithromycin	B	Standard indications
Bedaquiline	B	Not teratogenic in animals, but no human data. Use in MDRTB/XDRTB
Caspofungin	C	Embryotoxic in rodents; no human experience
Cidofovir	C	Teratogenic in animals (black box warning); risk in women unknown
Ciprofloxacin	C	Arthropathy in beagle dogs; not recommended in pregnancy but > 400 cases of use with no arthropathy or birth defects
Clarithromycin	C	Teratogenic in animals; increased rate of abortions in women; azithromycin preferred for MAC
Clindamycin	B	Standard indications
Clotrimazole troche	C	No complications expected with oral or vaginal use
Dapsone	C	Limited experience; may increase risk of kernicterus
Doxycycline	D	Risk to infant teeth and bones; avoid
Entecavir	C	Not teratogenic in rodents; no human data
Erythromycin	B	Standard indications
Ethambutol	C	Teratogenic at high doses in animal studies, appears safe in humans
Famciclovir	B	Limited data in humans; reserve for severe herpes
Fluconazole	C*	Bone defects in animals; reserve for severe and established fungal infections; Ampho B often preferred
Flucytosine	C	Bone defects in animals; use only after first trimester
Foscarnet	C	Teratogenic in animals and no data in humans; use for disseminated CMV

* Fluconazole is Class C for a single dose; Class D for multiple doses

TABLE 42: Drugs for Opportunistic Infections in Pregnancy
(cont.)

Agent	Class*	Recommendation
Ganciclovir	C	Teratogenic in animals; limited but favorable experience in humans
Interferon	C	Delay treatment until after pregnancy
INH	C	Standard indications + pyridoxine
Itraconazole	C	Teratogenic in animals and concern for azoles in pregnancy; use for systemic mycosis; Ampho B often preferred
Mefloquine	C	May increase risk of stillbirth
Metronidazole	B	Extensive favorable experience in pregnant women; standard indications
Paromomycin	C	Not absorbed; fetal toxicity unlikely
Pentamidine	C	Embryocidal in animals; limited experience in women
Primaquine	C	Limited experience; theoretical risk of hemolytic anemia with G6PD deficiency
Posaconazole	C	Teratogenic in animals; risk in women unknown
Pyrazinamide	C	Not teratogenic in rodents; limited experience in humans
Pyrimethamine	C	Teratogenic in rodents; limited human experience suggests risk of birth defect; if used, add leucovorin
Ribavirin	X	Teratogenic in animals; contraindicated in pregnancy
Rifabutin	B	Not teratogenic in animals
Rifampin	C	Teratogenic in animals; indicated for TB; Reports of neonatal haemorrhage; give vitamin K to mother and newborn at birth.
Sulfadiazine	C	Possible kernicterus if used near delivery
Telbivudine	B	Not teratogenic in rodents; limited data in humans
Valacyclovir	B	See acyclovir
Voriconazole	D	Teratogenic in rodents; Ampho B preferred

* Classes:
  A controlled studies show no risk
  B no evidence of risk in humans
  C risk not ruled out
  D positive evidence of risk
  X contraindicated in pregnancy

OPPORTUNISTIC INFECTIONS

Guidelines for the Prevention and Treatment of Opportunistic Infections in HIV-Infected Adults and Adolescents. 2018. https://aidsinfo.nih.gov/guidelines/html/4/adult-and-adolescent-oi-prevention-and-treatment-guidelines/0

TABLE 43: Guidelines for Prevention of Opportunistic Infections** (2017 NIH/CDC/IDSA Guidelines)

Infection/Organism	Indication	First Choice
Strongly Recommended		
Pneumocystis jirovecii	• CD4 < 200/mm³ or • CD4% < 14%, thrush, hx of AIDS defining illness or FUO • CD4 <250/mm³ if q 3 months monitoring not possible	• TMP-SMX 1 DS/d* or • TMP-SMX 1 SS/d*
Mycobacterium tuberculosis	See Page 92 for latent or active TB and HIV Co-infection	
Toxoplasma gondii	+ anti-Toxoplasma IgG positive and CD4 < 100/mm³	• TMP-SMX 1 DS* qd
Mycobacterium avium complex	• CD4 < 50/mm³	• Azithromycin 1200 mg/wk or 600 mg po 2x/wk or • Clarithromycin 500 mg bid† • Azithromycin 600 mg 2x/week
Varicella zoster	<u>Post-exposure</u> Chickenpox / shingles exposure and susceptible (no history of disease and varicella seronegative)	• VZIG 5 vials (6.25 mL) 125 IU/10 kg (max 625 IU) IM • Treat ASAP within 96 h post exposure preferred. Should be within 10 days.
	<u>Pre-exposure</u> No history of chickenpox, shingles, vaccine, or positive serology and CD4 count > 200/mm³	• Primary varicella vaccine (Varivax) (0.5 mL SQ) 2 doses 3 months apart

* SS= Single strength tablet, DS=Double strength tablet
**Prophylaxis against coccidioidomycosis, histoplasmosis, malaria, and penicilliosis only recommended with prolong exposure in endemic regions.
† Dose adjusted for concurrent PI or COBI with or without CrCL <30 ml/min.

Alternatives	Comments
• Dapsone 100 mg/d or 50 mg bid or • Dapsone 50 mg/d (or dapsone 200 mg/week) PLUS pyrimethamine 50 mg/wk + leucovorin 25 mg/wk or • Aerosol pentamidine 300 mg by Respigard II nebulizer once a month or • Atovaquone 1500 mg +/- pyrimethamine 25 mg + leucovorin 10 mg/d or • TMP-SMX 1 DS* 3x/wk	• Discontinue prophylaxis if CD4 > 200/mm^3 for > 3 mos • Restart prophylaxis if CD4 decreases to < 200/mm^3 • Pyrimethamine regimens for toxoplasmosis prophylaxis • TMP-SMX 1DS/d provides toxoplasmosis prophylaxis • Avoid dapsone with G6PD deficiency
• TMP-SMX 1 SS* qd or 1 DS 3x/week • Dapsone 50 mg/d + pyrimethamine 50 mg/wk + leucovorin 25 mg/wk • Dapsone 200 mg/wk + pyrimethamine 75 mg/wk + leucovorin 25 mg/wk • Atovaquone 1500 mg (± pyrimethamine 25 mg + leucovorin 10 mg)/d	• Discontinue prophylaxis if CD4 > 200/mm^3 for ≥ 3 mos • Restart prophylaxis if CD4 decreases to < 100-200/mm^3 • Repeat toxo serology if baseline serology negative and CD4 count subsequently declines to < 100/mm^3
• Rifabutin [†] 300 mg/d (adjust dose for concurrent ART)	• Discontinue prophylaxis if CD4 > 100/mm^3 for > 3 mos • Restart prophylaxis if CD4 decreases to < 50/mm^3 • Rule out active MAC before giving monotherapy prophylaxis
• VZIG treatment IND 1-800-843-7477 • Acyclovir 800 mg 5x/d or valacyclovir 1 g Q8h x 5-7 days can be considered (no data)	• Treat primary varicella infections with valacyclovir 1 gm TID or famciclovir 500 mg TID x 5-7 days. Give IV acyclovir 10 mg/kg IV q8h x7-10d for severe disease • Varicella vaccine should be given > 72 hrs after last dose of antiviral. • Vaccinate household contacts to prevent transmission to susceptible HIV+ patient
	• Routine serology not recommended • If vaccine causes disease, treat with acyclovir

TABLE 44: CDC/OI Guidelines for Vaccines in HIV-Infected Patients*

Infection/Organis	Indication	First Choice
Generally Recommended		
S. pneumoniae	• All patients with HIV regardless of CD4 count and no pneumococcal vaccine in 5 yrs • Consider if CD4 < 200/mm³	PCV 13 (Prevnar 13) 0.5 mL x 1, then PPSV23 (Pneumovax) 0.5 mL IM or SC ≥ 8 weeks later, then in 5 years. (MMWR 2012 61(40): 816) If prior PPSV23, PCV 13 ≥1 year later, then a second dose PPSV23 ≥ 8 weeks later, then in 5 years (Prevnar 13 $169.11/dose) (Pneumovax $86.71)
Hepatitis B	Susceptible (anti-HBc or anti-HBs negative) and HBsAg negative	Heplisav-B 0.5mL IM 2 doses (seperated by 1 month ($115/dose) OR Engerix-B 0.5mL IM 20 mcg/mL Dose at 0, 1 and 6 mo ($57.25/dose)
Influenza	All patients annually regardless of CD4 count (seasonal)	Inactivated influenza vaccine 0.5 mL IM ($15-21/dose)
Hepatitis A	Susceptible (anti-HAV negative) and risk (IDU, MSM, travel) or chronic liver disease (HBV or HCV infection); persons receiving clotting factor concentrate.	• Hepatitis A vaccine series: 1.0 mL x 2 at 0 and 6-12 mos (Havrix) ($64.21/dose) • Some delay until CD4 is > 200/mm³
Human papilloma virus (HPV)	Females and males, ages 11-12 yrs; 13-26 if unvaccinated. MSM, ages: up to age 26 Immunocompromised persons (HIV)-up to age 26	9 valent HPV vaccine (Gardasil 9) (6, 11, 16, 18, 31, 33, 45, 52, 58) 0.5 mL IM at 0, 1-2, and 6 month ($217.11/dose)
Tetanus diphtheria and acellular pertussis (Tdap) Tetanus and diphtheria (Td)	Female and males age 13-26	Single dose Tdap to all adults > 19 yrs who have not received Tdap ($39.35), then Td ($23.93) every 10 years.
Zoster	Age > 60 yrs and CD4 > 200/mm³	Preferred: Shingrix (0.5 mL IM ($140) x 2 doses 2-6 months apart) Alt:Zostavax 0.65 mL SQ ($212.66) x 1 dose
Varicella	Contraindicated with CD4 < 200/mm³	Varivax 0.5 mL SQ ($115.16) x 2 doses 4-8 weeks apart.
Meningococcal Conjugate Vaccine	All persons aged ≥ 2 months	Menactra 4 mcg/0.5mL ($112.93) Menveo 4 mcg/0.5mL ($117.49) Primary series: 2 doses 8-12 weeks apart. If previously vaccinated: 2nd dose > 8wks later. Booster q 5 years

* Recommendations are based on ACIP (CDC) 2015 (http://www.cdc.gov/vaccines/schedules/downloads/adult/adult-combined-schedule.pdf); Aberg J et al Primary Care Guideline for Management of Persons with HIV infection CID 2014; 58: e1; and Rubin LG et al 2013 IDSA Clinical Practice Guideline for Vaccination of the Immunocompromised Host CID 2013.

Alternatives	Comments
Pneumovax	Consider reimmunization if CD4 increases to > 200/mm³ and initial immunization was given when CD4 < 200/mm³ OR wait for CD4 count >200/mm3 before giving pneumovax.
None	Measure anti-HBs at one month after 3rd dose; if < 10 IU/mL: revaccinate w/ higher dose Engerix-B 40 mcg/mL (x 3 or 4 doses at 0, 1, 2, 6 month) or delay until CD4 count higher or use Heplisav-B (higher immunogenicity) Vaccination best when done w/ CD4 >350/mm³
Oseltamivir 75 mg qd	FluMist (live virus vaccine) contraindicated regardless of CD4 count.
None	Determine antibody response 1 mo post-vaccination; if negative, revaccinate. HCV co-infected patient should be vaccinated. Give ≥ 2 weeks prior to travel. Consider Hep A + B (Twinrix) 1 ml in 3 doses (0, 1, and 6 mo) only for HAV and HBV non-immune.
	If vaccination completed with quadrivalent or bivalent vaccine, may consider additional vaccination with 9 valent vaccine (no data). 9 valent vaccine (Gardasil 9) adds protection against five additional HPV types—31, 33, 45, 52 and 58.
	Tetanus prophylaxis in wound care: <3 prior doses or unknown vaccination, > 10 yrs post Td or severe injury >5 yrs
None	Revaccination with Shingrix may be considered in patients >70 yo who previously received Zostavax. Varicella vaccine (Varivax 2 doses separated 1-2 months apart) may be considered in VZV-seronegative adults with CD4 count > 200 /mm³ Susceptible patients (no Hx of varicella zoster and/or seronegative) should receive varicella immune globulin (VariZig) ASAP (within 10d of exposure to VZV).
	Meningococcal conjugate vaccine that covers serogroups A,C,W, and Y recommended MenACWY recommended for pts aged ≥ 56 years. If < 7 yo at previous dose, give first booster at 3 years then q5 thereafter. MenB vaccination in asplenic

Prices reported by private sector to CDC http://www.cdc.gov/vaccines/programs/vfc/awardees/vaccine-management/price-list/

TABLE 45: Treatment of Opportunistic Infections (NIH/CDC/IDSA)

Infection/Organism	Treatment
Bartonella	Bacillary angiomatosis, peliosis hepatitis, bacteremia, and osteomyelitis: Erythromycin 500 mg qid po or IV x ≥ 3 mos or doxycycline 100 mg bid po or IV x ≥ 3 mos Alternative: Azithromycin 500 mg po/d x ≥ 3 mos or clarithromycin 500 mg bid po x ≥ 3 mos CNS or severe infections: Doxycycline 100 mg po or IV q12h +/- rifampin 300 mg po q12h or IV > 3 mos
Candida: Thrush	Initial episode: Fluconazole 100 mg po x 7-14 d Fluconazole refractory: Itraconazole soln 200 mg/d po, posaconazole soln 400 mg bid po, amphotericin 0.3 mg/kg/d IV, anidulafungin 100 mg IV then 50 mg/d, caspofungin 50 mg/d IV, micafungin 150 mg/d IV or ampho B susp 100 mg/mL 1 mL qid (must be compounded by pharmacy)
Candida: Esophagitis	Preferred: Fluconazole 100-200 mg (up to 400-800 mg/d) po or IV x 14-21d or itraconazole 200 mg po daily x 14-21d Fluconazole refractory: Posaconazole soln 400 mg bid po x 28 d, ampho B 0.3-0.7 mg/kg/d IV or lipid ampho B 3-4 mg/kg/d, anidulafungin 100 mg IV then 50 mg/d IV, micafungin 150 mg/d IV, caspofungin 50 mg IV/d or voriconazole 200 mg bid po or IV
Candida: Vaginitis	Preferred: Fluconazole 150 mg po x 1 or topical azole x 3-7 d Recurrent or complicated: Fluconazole 100-200 mg daily or topical azole ≥ 7 d
Cryptosporidium	Preferred: ART to achieve CD4 > 100/mm³; antimotility agents and IV hydration Alternative (use in combination with ART): Nitazoxanide 0.5-1.0 gm po bid w/ food x 2 wks or paromomycin 500 mg po qid x 14-21 days.
Cryptococcal Meningitis, diffuse pulmonary cryptococcal disease, and severe extrapulmonary cryptococcal disease.	Preferred: Induction with liposomal amphotericin 3-4 mg/kg IV (or Ampho B 0.7 mg/kg/d) plus flucytosine 25 mg/kg qid po ≥ 2 wks then consolidation therapy with fluconazole 400 mg qd ≥ 8 wks, then maintenance therapy 200 mg/d for ≥ 12 months. Alternative induction: • 5FC 25mg/kg qid PLUS Ampho Lipid complex 5mg/kg x ≥ 2 wks • Fluconazole 800 mg daily PLUS [Ampho B 0.7-1mg/kg/d IV OR Liposomal Ampho 3-4 mg/kg] x ≥ 2 wks • Fluconazole 400-800 mg/d po or IV + flucytosine 25 mg/kg qid • Fluconazole 1200 mg PO or IV qd x ≥ 2 wks Alternative-consolidation: Itraconazole 200 mg po bid x 8 wks (less effective) Alternative-maintenance: Itraconazole 200 mg/d is less effective than fluconazole and can not be recommended. • For non-CNS cryptococcosis with mild-to-moderate symptoms, use fluconazole 400 mg PO daily x 12 months

(continued)

Comment
• May need long-term suppression with doxycycline or macrolide if relapse until CD4> 200 cells/mm^3 • Bartonella Endocarditis: Doxycycline 100 mg IV q12h + Gentamicin 1mg/kg q8h (or rifampin 300 mg IV or PO q12h x 2 weeks, then doxycycline 100 mg po q12h x 3-4 months. • May have severe Jarisch-Herxheilmer reaction in first 48 h
• Treat until CD4 > 200 cells for $\geq$ 6 months after 3-4 mo of treatment.
• Alternative: topical clotrimazole troches 10 mg po 5x/d; miconazole mucoadhesive buccal 50 mg tab once daily; nystatin susp 5 mL qid or as 1-2 flavored pastilles 4-5x/d x 7-14 days • Alternative systemic initial therapy: Itraconazole soln 200 mg/d po x 7-14 days or posaconazole oral suspension 400 mg po bid x 1d, then 400 mg po once daily x 7-14 days.
• Suppressive therapy: Indicated for severe or frequent reoccurrences; fluconazole 100 mg/d or itraconazole soln 200 mg/d. Discontinue when CD4 > 200/mm^3.
• Alternative initial therapy: Treat 14-21 d with voriconazole, isavuconazole, caspofungin, micafungin, anidulafungin (prior designated doses) or ambisome B 3-4 mg/kg/d IV or Ampho B 0.6 mg/kg/d. These alternative are generally used for fluconazole-refractory cases. • Suppressive therapy: Indicated for severe or frequent reoccurrences fluconazole 100-200 mg po or posaconazole 400 mg bid po Note: Fluconazole refractory cases that responded to echinocandins may be transitioned to oral voriconazole or posaconazole prophylaxis
• Alternative initial therapy: Itraconazole soln 200 mg/d po x 3-7 d • Maintenance (for severe or frequent reoccurrences): Fluconazole 150 mg po q wk
Antimotility agents: tincture of opium may be more effective than loperamide.
Lactase deficiency common due to diarrhea. Avoid milk product
• High opening pressure: LP to drain CSF until 50% OP. Repeat daily until OP < 200 mm Hg (this is critical). CSF shunting may be needed if OP is not under control with daily LP. • Patients given 5FC should have blood levels measured to assure 2 h post dose level is 25-100 mg/L (after 3-5 doses). Adjust dose for renal failure (see page 114). • Lipid amphotericin is preferred over ampho B due to equivalent efficacy and lower rate of nephrotoxicity and infusion reactions. • Addition of flucytosine to ampho B increases rate of CSF clearance of cryptococcus, lower relapse rates, and a trend toward improved survial. • > 2 weeks induction recommended if PT has not clinically improved, with persistent $\uparrow$ ICP, and has positive CSF cultures at 2 weeks • After induction and consolidation phase, treat with fluconazole for at least a year, remains asymptomatic, and until CD4 count $\geq$ 100/mm^3 for >3 mos and VL <50 • Continue fluconazole maintenance lifelong or reinitiate fluconazole if CD4 <100/mm^3 • Delay initiation of ART until after 2-10 weeks of induction/consolidation antifungal. Earlier initiation may be considered in pts with severe immunosuppression (CD4 <50/mm^3). • Some experts recommend short course corticosteroid only for management of severe IRIS.

(continued)

TABLE 45: Treatment of Opportunistic Infections (cont.)

Infection/Organism	Treatment
Cytomegalovirus: Retinitis	Preferred for vision-threatening lesion (within 1500 micron of the fovea): Intravitreal ganciclovir (2mg) or foscarnet (2.4mg) x 1 to 4 doses over 7-10 days + valganciclovir 900 mg bid x 14-21 d, then 900 mg qd Preferred for peripheral lesions: Oral valganciclovir 900 mg bid po x 14-21 d, then 900 mg qd Alternatives systemic treatment: • Ganciclovir 5 mg/kg bid IV x 14 -21d, then 5 mg/kg/d IV, or • Foscarnet 60 mg/kg q8h IV or 90 mg/kg q12h IV x 14-21 d, then 90-120 mg/kg IV qd, or • Cidofovir 5 mg/kg q7d IV x 2 doses, then 5 mg/kg q14d IV
Cytomegalovirus: Colitis, Esophagitis, Pneumonia	Preferred: ganciclovir (IV) per above doses for CMV retinitis x 21-42 d or until symptoms resolution. Switch to valganciclovir (oral) once PO can be tolerated. Alternative: foscarnet (IV) per above doses Maintenance: Role is unclear; consider after relapse
Cytomegalovirus: Neurologic Disease	Preferred: Ganciclovir + foscarnet per above doses for CMV retinitis Maintenance: IV foscarnet + po valganciclovir for life. initiate ART ASAP.
Hepatitis B Virus (HBsAg+≥ 6 mos)	Treatment for HIV/HBV at least 2 agents active versus both viruses (usually TDF/FTC or TAF/FTC) • 3TC/FTC-naive: TAF/FTC 25/200mg/d or TDF/FTC 300/200 mg/d + additional agent for HIV • 3TC/FTC-experienced + detectable HBV DNA (assume 3TC/FTC/telbivudine resistance): ○ Add TDF 300 mg qd + (3TC/FTC) or entecavir 1 mg/d (use only if HIV viral load is undetectable) Duration: Both treated indefinitely Treat HBV and not HIV: Treat with Peg-interferon 180 mcg weekly x 48 week if elevated ALT, and HBV DNA >2000 IU/mL, significant liver fibrosis, advanced liver disease, or cirrhosis.
Hepatitis C Virus	See Table 52. Treatment of HCV
Histoplasmosis	• For less severe disease without CNS involvement: Itraconazole 200 mg PO TID x 3 days, then 200 mg PO BID x ≥ 12 months. • Preferred treatment for non-CNS moderately severe to severe disease: Liposomal ampho 3mg/kg IV daily x 4-6 wks, then itraconazole 200 mg po BID to TID (target random itraconazole level > 1 mcg/mL) x ≥ 12 months and until resolution of abnormal CSF findings. • Preferred treatment for CNS disease: Liposomal ampho 5mg/kg IV daily x ≥ 2 wks, then itraconazole 200 mg po BID x ≥ 12 months (and until resolution of CNS symptoms). • Long-term suppression with itraconazole 200 mg daily recommended in patients with severe disease and/or CNS involvement OR relapse with appropriate therapy.

- Ganciclovir preferred over foscarnet and cidofovir due to lower rates of toxicities.
- Duration of Systemic treatment: Continue until inactive disease + CD4 > 100/mm^3 x 3-6 mos Every 3 months ophthalmology F/U required. Reinitiate maintenance therapy if CD4 count < 100 cells/mm^3.
- ART critical component of treatment
- Immune recovery uveitis: Periocular steroids or short course oral prednisone.
- Intraocular ganciclovir implant no longer available
- 1L saline hydration before cidofovir infusion. Give probenecid 2gm 3hrs prior and 1gm given 2hrs and 8hrs after cidofovir infusion.

- Maintenance: Consider after relapse or severe disease
- CMV pneumonia: Indications are CMV by histology plus lack of response to other pathogens
- ART: Critical component of treatment

- ART is critical.
- Prognosis pre-HAART was poor.

Indications to treat HBV:
  - Standard recommendations for treating HBV: abnormal ALT + HBeAg pos + HBV DNA > 20,000 IU/mL OR abnormal ALT + HBV DNA > 2,000 IU/mL with HBeAg neg
  - The need to treat HIV (with HIV/HBV active drugs)

If HIV-coinfected and not receiving ART, treatment of HBV with the following agents can result in HIV resistance: 3TC, FTC, TDF, TAF, telbivudine, adefovir and entecavir. Avoid

- HIV/HCV/HBV co-infection: Treat HIV/HBV/HCV
- When changing HIV agents: Maintain agents active against HBV
- Discontinuation of anti-HBV agents: May cause life-threatening flare - restart
- Telbivudine/FTC/3TC: Assume cross-resistance

- Alternatives to Liposomal ampho: Ampho Lipid complex 3mg/kg/d OR Ampho cholesteryl sulfate complex 3mg/kg/d.

- Alternatives to itraconazole: voriconazole 400 mg PO BID x 1 day, then 200 mg BID OR Posaconazole 400 mg PO BID OR Fluconazole 800 mg daily.

- See table 16 (page 35) for drug-drug interactions with azole antifungals

- Monitor itraconazole concentrations. Target random serum concentrations >1 mcg/mL.

Infection/Organism	Treatment
Herpes Simplex: Mucocutaneous and Keratitis	<u>Mucocutaneous HSV</u> Preferred: Valacyclovir 1 gm po bid, acyclovir 400 mg po tid, famciclovir 500 mg po bid x 5-10 days for orolabial or genital lesions. Severe: Acyclovir 5 mg/kg IV q8h, then oral agent for $\geq$ 21 d <u>HSV Keratitis</u> Preferred: Trifluridine 1% ophthalmic soln 1 drop q2h up to 9 drops/d 10-21 days (plus corticosteroid for stromal keratitis)
Herpes Simplex: Encephalitis	Preferred: Acyclovir 10 mg/kg q8h IV x 14-21 d
Herpes Zoster	Acute localized dermatomal: Valacyclovir 1 gm po tid OR famciclovir 500 mg po q8h x 7-10 days (longer if lesions are slow to resolve). Extensive cutaneous lesions or visceral involvement: Acyclovir 10-15 mg/kg IV q8h until clinical improvement, then switch to PO valacyclovir.
Microsporidia	<u>Intestinal caused by E. bienuesi:</u> ART to get CD4 > 100/mm^3 + rehydration + antimotility agents + fumagillin 20 mg po tid or TNP-470 (not available in US). Nitazoxanide (minimal efficacy with low CD4 count Intestinal and disseminated (not occular) caused by Microsporidia (othe than E. bienuesi and V corneae): Albendazole 400 mg po bid + ART (. <u>Disseminated disease due to Trachipleistophora and Anncaliia:</u> Itraconazole 400 mg po qd + albendazole 400 mg bid plus ART. <u>Ocular Infections:</u> Fumagillin 70mcg/mL or Fumidil B 3mg/mL- use 2 gtt q2h x 4 days, then 2 gtts qid + ART until eye sx resolve and CD4 > 200/mm^3 x 6 mo.
Myobacterium avium Complex	Preferred: Clarithromycin 500 mg po bid + ethambutol 15 mg/kg qd OR azithromycin 500-600 mg po qd + ethambutol 15 mg/kg po qd Adding a third/fourth drug should be considered w/ severe disease, CD4 50/mm^3, or abscence of effective ART. • rifabutin* 300 mg po qd • ciprofloxacin 500-750 mg bid po, levofloxacin 500 mg qd po, or moxifloxacin 400 mg qd po or • amikacin 10-15 mg/kg qd IV or streptomycin 1 gm IM/d
Mycobacterium tuberculosis	See Tables 48-51
Pneumocystis jirovecii	**Preferred:** • TMP-SMX (15-20 mg/kg/d TMP and 75-100 mg SMX/kg/d) q6-8h IV; switch to po when clinically improved or • TMP-SMX 2 DS tid (TMP 5 mg/kg tid) x 21 d (for 70 Kg patient) Alternative - severe disease: • Pentamidine 4 mg/kg/d IV infused over > 60 min • Primaquine 30 mg po/d** + clindamycin 600-900 mg IV q8h or 450 mg po q6 x 21 days Alternative - mild or moderate disease: • Dapsone** 100 mg qd +TMP 5 mg/kg tid x 21 d; or • Primaquine** 30 mg base qd + clindamycin 450 mg po q6h x 21 d, or • Atovaquone 750 mg bid po with food x 21 d (less effective)

* Rifabutin reduces levels of clarithromycin by 50% (consider azithromycin if rifabutin is used). Rifabutin may need dose adjustment based on ART regimen.

Acyclovir-resistant HSV: Foscarnet 80-120 mg/kg/d IV in 2-3 daily doses; IV cidofovir 5mg/kg
Alternative for acyclovir-resistant HSV: Topical trifluridine (compounded with ophthalmic solutions), topical cidofovir (compounded with IV cidofovir), or topical imiquimod x 21-28 days
Chronic suppressive treatment: valacyclovir 500 mg bid, acyclovir 400 mg bid, or famciclovir 500 mg bid for severe HSV recurrences
ARVs may decrease severity of HSV episodes

Inadequate CSF concentrations with PO valacyclovir.

VZV progressive outer retinal necrosis: IV ganciclovir +/- IV foscarnet + intravitreal ganciclovir +/- intravitreal foscarnet (consult ophthalmology)
VZV acute retinal necrosis: IV acyclovir 10-15 mg/kg q8h x 10-14 d + intravitreal ganciclovir 2mg/0.05mL 2x/week x 1-2 doses, then valacyclovir 1g TID x 6 weeks (consult ophthalmology)

Nitazoxanide has minimal efficacy against E. bienuesi in pts with low CD4 count.

Treat until no signs and symptoms of microsporidiosis and CD4 >200/mm^3 x 6 mos.

Duration: Until MAC treatment ≥ 12 mos, asymptomatic and CD4 count > 100/mm^3 x 6 mos. Reinitiate secondary prophylaxis w/ CD4 <100/mm3
Test susceptibility to clarithromycin and azithromycin (especially with clinical failure).
NSAIDs for symptoms attributed to IRIS; use 20-40 mg prednisone x 4-8 weeks if IRIS symptoms persist
Use azithromycin to minimize CYP3A4 drug-drug interactions.

For CD4 < 50 cells/mm^3: Initiate ART within 2 weeks of TB treatment
for CD4 = or > 50 cells/mm^3: ART can be delayed 2-4 weeks, but should initiate within 8 weeks of TB treatment. Some experts recommend early ART (within 2-4 wks) in severe HIV
Hypoxia (Pa0$_2$ < 70 mm Hg or A-a O$_2$ gradient > 35 mm Hg): Start steroid ASAP (within 72h). Prednisone: 40 mg bid days 1-5, 40 mg qd days 6-10, then 20 mg qd days 11-21, or IV methylprednisolone as 75% prednisone dose.
Failure to respond:
Use alternative regimen but note that initial response is usually slow (e.g. > 5 d)
Sulfa allergy: see page 89 for sulfa desensitization protocol. TMP/SMX can be considered if no hx of SJS or TEN.
Secondary Prophylaxis:
TMP-SMX 1 DS once daily or TMP-SMX 1 SS once daily (preferred)
Dapsone 100 mg/d OR dapsone 50 mg/d + pyrimethamine 50 mg/wk + leucovorin 25 mg/wk
Dapsone 200 mg/week + pyrimethamine 75 mg/wk + leucovorin 25 mg/wk
Aerosol pentamidine 300 mg once per month by Respigard II nebulizer or
Atovaquone 1500 mg +/- pyrimethamine 25 mg/d + leucovorin 10 mg/d

* Primaquine or dapsone: screening for G6PD recommended.

TABLE 45: Treatment of Opportunistic Infections (cont.)

Infection/Organism	Treatment
Salmonella	**Preferred:** Ciprofloxacin 500-750 mg po (or 400 mg IV) q12h Alternative (if susceptible): • Moxifloxacin 400 mg po or IV q24h • Levofloxacin 750 mg po or IV q24h • TMP-SMX 160/800 mg po or IV q12h, or • Ceftriaxone 1 gm IV q24h, **or** Cefotaxime 1gm IV q8h
Shigella	**Preferred:** Ciprofloxacin 500-750 mg po (or 400 mg IV) q12h Alternative (if susceptible):Alternative (if susceptible): • Moxifloxacin 400 mg po or IV q24h • Levofloxacin 750 mg po or IV q24h • TMP-SMX 160/800 mg po or IV q12h, or • Azithromycin 500 mg po q24h (x 5 days)
Toxoplasma gondii	**Preferred - acute phase** (treat for at least 6 wks): Pyrimethamine 200 mg x 1 po, then 50 mg (< 60 kg) or 75 mg (> 60 kg) qd po + sulfadiazine 1 g (< 60 kg) or 1.5 g (> 60 kg) qid po + leucovorin 10-25 mg qd po x ≥ 6 wks. Continue longer if clinical or radiologic effect i extensive or response is delayed. Alternative - acute: • Pyrimethamine + leucovorin (as above) PLUS clindamycin 600 g q6h po or IV (preferred) • Pyrimethamine + leucovorin +Atovaquone 1500 mg bid po with food • TMP-SMX 5 mg/kg bid IV or po, **or** • Atovaquone 1.5 g bid po with food PLUS sulfadiazine 1-1.5 g po q6h • Atovaquone 1.5 g bid po • Atovaquone 1.5 g bid po PLUS pyrimethamine (as above) **Preferred - maintenance phase** (after ≥ 6 wk initial treatment): • Pyrimethamine 25-50 mg/d po + sulfadiazine 2-4 gm po/d in 2-4 doses + leucovorin 10-25 mg/d Alternative - maintenance: • Pyrimethamine 25-50 mg/d + leucovorin 10-25 mg po/d + clindamycin 600 mg q8h po • Atovaquone 750-1500 mg po q12h PLUS [pyrimethamine 25 mg po qd and leucovorin 10 mg po/d] • Atovaquone 750-1500 mg po 12h + sulfadiazine 1-2 gm q12h • TMP/SMX 1DS po q12h or TMP/SMX 1 DS q24h (*consider if pt <60kg) • Atovaquone 750-1500 mg po 12h

* added by author

Comment

- All HIV-infected pts should be treated due to increase risk of bacteremia (20-100 fold) and mortality (up to 7-fold)
- Mild gastroenteritis only and CD4 > 200/mm³: Treat 7-14 d; if CD4 count < 200/mm³: Treat 2-6 wks
- Gastroenteritis w/ bacteremia: 1) CD4 >200/mm3, treat for 14d (treat longer if complicated e.g. metastatic bone foci) 2) CD4 < 200/mm3, treat for 2-6 weeks.
- With recurrent gastroenteritis +/- bacteremia: consider treatment until immune reconstitution (CD4 > 200/mm³ and VL < 50 c/mL)

- Consider withholding abx if CD4 >500 cells/mm3 and diarrhea resolved prior to shigella culture confirmation.
- Duration of treatment
Gastroenteritis: 7-10 days (if azithromycin used treat for 5 days)
Bacteremia: a minimum of 14 days (azithromycin not recommended with bacteremia)
Recurrent infection: up to 6 weeks
- Increased fluoroquinolones resistance in US (associated with international travel, MSM, and homelessness. Do not use fluoroquinolones if ciprofloxacin MIC >0.12 mcg/mL even if the lab reports the isolate as sensitive.

- Acute phase should be extended >6 weeks if extensive disease or incomplete clinical/radiological response at 6 weeks.

- Adjunctive dexamethasone given only if mass effect (check for drug-drug interactions with ARVs)
- Anticonvulsants if history of seizures only. Check for drug-drug interactions between anticonvulsants and ARVs.

- Treat until free of signs and symptoms of toxo encephalitis and CD4 > 200/mm³ for > 6 months.

- Reinitiate maintenance if CD4 count < 200/mm³.

- If pyrimethamine unavailable, use TMP/SMX regimen. http://www.daraprimdirect.com for access information.

- Rapid desensitization protocol for patients with sulfa allergy: Time 0h TMP/SMX 0.004/0.2mg, Time 1h TMP/SMX 0.04/0.2mg, Time 2h TMP/SMX 0.4/2mg, Time 3h TMP/SMX 4/20 mg, Time 4 hr 40/200 mg, Time 5h TMP/SMX 160/800mg. Give atovaquone until full dose TMP/SMX can be given.

- Leucovorin may be increased to 50 mg daily or twice daily to reverse pyrimethamine associated ADR (e.g bone marrow suppression)

- Add PCP prophylaxis if on clindamycin + pyrimethamine.

TABLE 46: Immune Reconstitution Syndrome (IRIS)

Definition: MA French (CID 2004;18:1615)		
Must have major criteria A and B plus any two minor criteria		
Major Criteria		
A	Atypical presentation of an opportunistic infection or tumor in patients responding to ART • Localized disease with severe fever or pain • Exaggerated inflammatory response • Atypical inflammatory response such as necrosis, exaggerated granulomas, suppuration or perivascular lymphocytic local infiltrate • Progression or organ dysfunction or enlargement of preexisting lesion after definite improvement with pathogen specific treatment prior to ART plus exclusion of treatment toxicity and new alternative diagnosis	
B	HIV VL decrease > 1-log_{10} c/mL	
Minor Criteria		
• Increase CD4 count • Increase in immune response specific to the relevant pathogen such as skin test for TB • Spontaneous resolution of disease with ART and without disease-specific treatment		
Alternate Definition: Robertson, et al. (CID 2006 ;42 :1639)		
• New or worsening symptoms of an infection or inflammatory condition after starting ART PLUS • Symptoms not explained by newly acquired infection, predicted course of previously diagnosed condition or adverse drug effects • HIV VL decrease > 1-log_{10} c/mL		
OI	Clinical Features	Treatment/Comments
Common to all opportunistic infections	• Defined as a paradoxical worsening of a prior condition soon after starting ART • MAC and TB account for 30% of reported cases; less common with cryptococcal meningitis and CMV retinitis • Usually occurs at 1-8 wks post ART initiation • Baseline CD4 count is usually < $50/mm^3$ • Rapid reduction in HIV viral load • May occur while treating OI, at time of OI clinical stability or as newly detected OI	• Usual treatment is to continue ART, antimicrobial therapy agents for the OI, and give NSAIDs and/or steroids if severe IRIS • ACTG A5164 compared early ART (<14 days from OI dx) vs delayed (42-84 days). Early ART improved survival. • IRIS reportedly rare with: histoplasmosis, aspergillosis, bartonellosis, cryptosporidiosis, and Candida sp.

TABLE 47: Immune Reconstitution Syndrome

(Adapted from Clin Infect Dis 2004;38:1159 and 2016 DHHS Opportunistic Infection Guidelines)

Agent	Clinical Features	Treatment/Comments
M. avium complex	Focal adenitis with systemic IRIS simulating TB IRIS. Expression highly variable with adenitis, Other expressions-pulmonary infiltrates, liver granuloma, mediastinitis, osteomyelitis, cerebritis	• ART, antibiotics, ± NSAIDs or high dose steroids • Common cause of IRIS-10% of cases
M. tuberculosis	Hectic fevers, worsening adenopathy, new and worsening pulmonary infiltrates. Severe IRIS: enlarging cerebral tuberculomas, meningitis, pericardial effusions, extensive pulmonary lesions, splenomegaly. Incidence is 16% and fatality rate 3.2%. Other expression include ARDS, adenitis, hepatitis, renal failure, epididymitis	• ART, anti-TB meds, NSAIDS ± high dose steroids. • *Steroid dose for severe IRIS: With rifampin: prednisone 1.5mg/kg/d x 2 weeks, then 0.75mg/kg/d x 2 weeks. With rifabutin 1mg/kg/d x 2 weeks, then 0.5mg/kg/d x 2 weeks. • Slower taper (over months) may be required in some pts.
Cryptococcus	Worsening clinical meningitis despite microbiological response. Other expressions-palsy, hearing loss, abscess, mediastinitis, adenitis, fever, pneumonia, pleural effusion.	• Continue ART and antifungal therapy and reduce intracranial pressure if indicated. Some experts use of short course steroid. • ACTG A5164 favored early earlier ART, but some studies show worse outcome (see page 82).
P. jirovecii	Pneumonia	ART, anti-PCP meds, steroids
PML (JC virus)	IRIS possible in first wks or months of ART with CNS lesions showing contrast enhancement, edema and mass effect	High dose steroids (methylpred 1gm/d x 3-5d then prednisone 60mg/d with taper over 1-6 weeks. Contrast MRI at 2-6 weeks helpful.
HSV	Chronic erosive ulcers, encephalitis	ART, antivirals, steroids
Varicella zoster	Zoster flare	ART, antivirals
CMV	Retinitis-inflammation in anterior chamber or vitreous; can lead to vision loss. Cytoid macular edema, uveitis	ART, steroids + anti-CMV agents. Periocular, intravitreal, or systemic steroid administration all reported effective
KS	New onset KS or exacerbation of previously stable disease including tracheal mucosal edema, obstruction	ART +/- steroids
Hepatitis B	Hepatitis fare with elevated ALT and AST	ART active against HBV. Must distinguish ART-agent hepatotoxicity (or other causes), but need to discontinue ART is rare. Liver biopsy may show eosinophils (drug toxicity) or portal inflammation (viral hepatitis)
HPV	Inflamed warts	Steroids, surgery
HSV	Atypical mucocutaneous lesions refractory to HSV therapy (rare)	ART, antiviral
Toxoplasma	Encephalitis	ART, Steroids

**Pre-emptive steroid should be offered to high-risk pts w/ CD4 <100/mm3 and starting ART and TB Rx within 30 days.

TREATMENT OF TUBERCULOSIS (American Thoracic Society / Centers for Disease Control and Prevention /Infectious Diseases Society of America: Treatment of Tuberculosis CID Oct 2016 ; http://www.cdc.gov/tb/topic/treatment, and NIH/CDC/IDSA Updated Opportunistic Infections Guidelines, 2017)

TABLE 48: Latent TB and HIV Co-Infection

Candidates for tuberculosis skin test (TST)or interferon gamma release assay (IGRA):

- Screen with TST or IGRA. IGRA is preferred in patients with recent BCG.
- IGRA has comparable or better sensitivity and is more specific than TST, with less cross-reactivity with other mycobacteria. Immunodeficiency decreases sensitivity of all tests
- All HIV-infected patients without prior positive test upon entry into HIV care. If negative, retest once ART initiated adn CD4 >200/mm³
- Repeat testing annually for patients at risk for repeated/ongoing TB exposures
- All HIV-infected patients with prior negative skin test who are discovered to be contacts of pulmonary cases

Indications for treatment of latent tuberculosis infection

- Positive PPD (≥ 5 mm induration) or positive IGRA plus no prior completed treatment of latent or active TB. IGRA and TST may remain positive even after treatment
- Recent contact with infectious TB case should be considered for latent TB treatment. Contacts initially TST /IGRA negative should have test repeated 12 wks after last TB exposure. Clinical decision based on risk regarding completion of treatment or discontinuation if test negative at 12 wks.
- Rule out active TB based on symptoms, chest x-ray, Microbiological testing if inidcated(AFB smear, cultures, and Xpert) prior to initiation of latent TB treatment

Treatment of latent tuberculosis

- Preferred Regimens:
  1) INH 300 mg + pyridoxine 25 mg qd for 9 mos (270 doses in 12 mos); or
  2) INH 900 mg 2x/wk + pyridoxine 25 mg/d by directly observed therapy for 9 mos (76 doses in 12 mos)
- Alternative Regimens (with consideration of ARV drug interactions:
  - Rifampin 10 mg/kg (600 mg max) x 4 mos or
  - Rifabutin with dose adjustment based on ARV regimen x 4 mos
  - [Rifapentine 750mg (32.1-49.9kg) or 900 mg (≥ 50kg) + INH 900 mg (plus pyridoxine 50mg/d)] X3months Not recommended in HIV-infected patients on interacting ARVs (e.g PI/r, NNRTIs, EVG, DTG, TAF). Use RAL, EFV, TDF/FTC, ABC/3TC.
- MDR-TB Exposure: Expert consultation is recommended for persons who are likely to be infected with INH- and RIF- (multidrug) resistant-TB and at high risk of reactivation

Monitoring therapy

- See clinician monthly to review symptoms suggesting hepatitis
- LFTs (ALT and bilirubin) at baseline, at minimum repeat 1 mo, 3 mos, and with symptoms of hepatitis. D/C and consider alternative if asymptomatic and ALT increases to ≥ 5x ULN or if symptomatic and ALT increases to ≥ 3x ULN

TABLE 49: Treatment of Drug-Susceptible Active Tuberculosis†

Phase 1 (8 wks)	Phase 2 (4-7 mos)*: Regimen, Doses, Minimal Duration
PREFERRED INH, RIF, PZA, EMB 8 wks • 7 d/wk for 8 wks (56 doses); or • 5 d/wk for 8 wks (minimum 40 doses observed)**	PREFERRED • INH/RIF 7 d/wk for 18 wks (126 doses); or • INH/RIF 5 d/wk for 18 wks (minimum 90 doses observed)**
ALTERNATE INH, RIF, PZA, EMB 8 wks • 7 d/wk for 8 wks (56 doses); or • 5 d/wk for 8 wks w DOT (40 doses)	ALTERNATE • INH/RIF 3x/wk for 18 wks (54 doses)
INH, RIF, PZA, EMB 8 wks • 3 x/wk for 8 wks (24 doses)	USE WITH CAUTION • INH/RIF 3x/wk for 18 wks (54 doses)
IF PZA NOT TOLERATED INH, RIF, EMB 8 wks • 7 d/wk for 8 wks (56 doses); or • 5 d/wk for 8 wks (40 doses)	• INH/RIF 7 d/wk for 31 wks (217 doses); or • INH/RIF 5 d/wk for 31 wks (155 doses); or

INH = Isoniazid, RIF = Rifampin, PZA = Pyrazinamide, EMB = Ethambutol
* Patients with cavitation at baseline or positive cultures at 2 mos should receive 31 wks continuation phase for total of 9 mos. See Table 51 (page 94) for treatment durations for CNS, bone/joints.
**5d/wk has never been studied compared to 7d/wk. 5d/wk is a minimum target for observation
† Directly observed therapy (DOT) recommended for all patients with HIV-related active TB to document treatment completion of recommended # of doses. Note that total doses is considered more important than total duration.
Paucity of data on optimal duration. In ART-era, total 6 months likely effective. Older cohort studies have suggested therapy 8mo or longer had lower recurrence risk. Extend therapy if not on ART Intermittent regimens, poor adherence, and low drug concentrations have been associated with failure. Consider drug levels. Daily therapy in both intensive and continuation phase now preferred.

TABLE 50: Doses of Antituberculosis Drugs – First Line Drugs

Drug	5-7 daily per wk	2 x/wk	3 x/wk
INH*	5 mg/kg (300)*†	15 mg/kg (900)*†	15 mg/kg (900)*†
RIF*	10 mg/kg (600)*	10 mg/kg (600)*	10 mg/kg (600)*
PZA (wt) 40-55 kg 56-74 kg 76-90 kg	 1.0 gm 1.5 gm 2.0 gm	 2.0 gm 3.0 gm 4.0 gm	 1.5 gm 2.5 gm 3.0 gm
EMB (wt) 40-55 kg 56-74 kg 76-90 kg > 90 kg	 800 mg 1200 mg 1600 mg 1600 mg	 2000 mg 2800 mg 4000 mg 4000 mg	 1200 mg 2000 mg 2400 mg 2400 mg

* Usual dose in mg in parentheses.
† INH should be given with pyridoxine. Dose at 25 mg on each day INH is given.
Consider therapeutic drug level monitoring, particularly for rifamycin and isoniazid

TABLE 51: Special Considerations for TB Treatment with HIV Co-Infection

Special issues for TB/HIV co-infection

All HIV patients should have TB evaluation; all TB patients should be evaluated for HIV

Risk of active TB increases with decline in CD4 count, but the increase risk is noted early in HIV disease with the CD4 count is > 500/mm³

Always treat TB first and do not start concurrent therapy (unless advanced HIV) due to pill burden and overlapping toxicity (rash, hepatitis, GI intolerance)
- Timing of ART base of CD4 and disease severity (see below).

IRIS is common and is most frequent with a baseline CD4 < 100/mm³ and with treatment initiated in first 2 mos. Clinical features include high fevers, deceasing respiratory function, adenopathy, CNS lesions, and pleural effusions.
- IRIS treatment:non-steroidals if uncomplicated; Steroid for severe IRIS reactions.
  - Suggested steroid regimen with rifampin based regimen-Prednisone 1.5 mg/kg/d x 2 weeks, then 0.75 mg/kg/d x 2 weeks

Suggested steroid regimen with rifabutin based regimen-Prednisone 1.0 mg/kg/d x 2 weeks, then 0.5 mg/kg/d x 2 weeks

Adjunctive steroids improve survival with HIV-associated TB meningitis, with taper over 6-8 weeks. Steroids can be considered selectively in TB pericarditis in patients at risk for constriction (early constriction, large effusion), but not routinely.

Drug-drug Interactions between rifampin and rifapentine and ART:
- TDF, FTC, 3TC, ABC can be used with standard TB regimens. Recent data suggests TAF may be used with rifampin; RBT has not been studied.
- EFV-based ART can be given using standard regimens;RPV and ETR should not be used
- PI-based ART requires rifabutin (150mg once/daily) in place of rifampin (see p37)
- EVG/COBI/TDF/FTC, EVG/c/TAF/FTC, BIC/TAF/FTC-should be avoided with rifamycin
- DTG 50 mg BID or RAL 800 mg BID plus 2NRTIs can be used with rifampin; both can be used at standard doses with RBT

Duration of treatment

- Intensive phase: 2 mos-INH/(RIF or RBT)/EMB/PZA with discontinuation of EMB if strain is pan-sensitive. Daily therapy (7d/wk) is preferred. Consider TB drug levels
- Continuation phase: INH/(RIF or RBT). Daily therapy is preferred.
- Total duration
  - Pulmonary TB without cavity and neg sputum at 2 mo: 6 mo
  - Pulmonary TB + cavity or positive sputum at 2 mo: 9 mo
  - Extrapulmonary TB with CNS involvement: 9-12 mos
  - Extrapulmonary TB with bone or joint involvement: 6-9 mos
  - Extrapulmonary TB at other sites without CNS, bone, or joint involvement: 6 mos

Timing of starting ART with TB/HIV (2016 DHHS Guidelines; 2016 WHO Guidelines)

- CD4 < 50: Start ART within 2 weeks of starting TB treatment
- CD4 ≥ 50: ART can be delayed 2-4 wks but should be started by wk 8 of TB treatment

Some experts recommend starting ART within 2-4 wks in pts with CD4 ≥ 50 and severe HIV disease. Consider delaying ART with TB meningitis beyond 2wks

TABLE 52: Treatment of Hepatitis C:

(Amer Assoc for Study of Liver Diseases (AALSD) and Infectious Disease Society of America (IDSA)
(http://www.hcvguidelines.org)

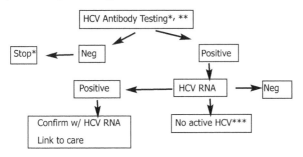

*Risk for HCV: Birth cohort: Born between 1945-1965 or other risk factor: IDU, hemodialysis, healthcare risk injury from HCV source, transfusion, organ transplant before 1992, or clotting factor concentrates before 1987, incarceration, HIV infection, unexplained liver disease, solid organ donor
**Annual testing for IDUs, HIV-infected MSM with unprotected sex
*** Retest Ab or HCV RNA recommended if risk within the past 6 months.

Active HCV infection

1) Patient education concerning transmission risks; 2) patient should avoid ETOH; 3) Evaluate for concurrent hepatic risks-HBV and HIV serology; 4) Vaccinate for HAV and HBV if not immune

Evaluation

Evaluate for fibrosis: Liver biopsy, Fibroscan, or non-invasive biomarkers

Evaluation by a practitioner who can provide comprehensive care including antiviral HCV therapy.

HBV reactivation has been observed during HCV treatment with interferon free regimens. HBV testing and treatment recommended. See page 61 and 84 for HBV treatment.

Goal of Treatment

Sustained viral response, i.e cure

Candidates for Treatment

All HCV infected patients can benefit from treatment

Highest Priorities for HCV treatment: 1) Advanced fibrosis (metavir F3) or compensated cirrhosis [metavir F4]) 2) Organ transplant 3) Type 2 or 3 essential mixed cryoglobulinemia with end organ involvement (vasculitis) 4) Proteinuria, nephrosis, or membranoproliferative glomerulonephritis

High Priorities for HCV treatment due to high risk of complications: HIV-coinfection, metavir F2, HBV co-infection, additional source of liver disease (eg NASH, debilitating fatigue, type2 insulin resistant diabetes, porphyria cutanea tarda

Priority based on elevated risk of HCV transmission: High risk MSM, active IDU, incarcerated persons, long term hemodialysis, women with child-bearing potential desiring pregnancy, healthcare workers who perform invasive procedures.

TABLE 52: Treatment of Hepatitis C:

(Amer Assoc for Study of Liver Diseases (AALSD) and Infectious Disease Society of America (IDSA) (http://www.hcvguidelines.org accessed 11/03/2018)

Treatment naive w/ genotype 1a

1) Daily fixed-dose combination Mavyret [glecaprevir (300mg)/pibrentasvir (120mg) x8 weeks (no cirrhosis) or x12 weeks (compensated cirrhosis).

2) Daily fixed-dose combination Harvoni [ledipasvir (90 mg) + sofosbuvir (400 mg)] x12 weeks in pts without cirrhosis or compensate cirrhosis. For pts who are non-black, HIV negative, and HCV RNA vial load <6 million IU/mL treat for 8 weeks.

3) Daily fixed-dose combination Epclusa [sofosbuvir (400 mg)/velpatasvir (100 mg)] x 12 weeks in patients without cirrhosis or compensated cirrhosis)

4) Daily fixed-dose combination Zepatier [elbasvir (50 mg)/grazoprevir (100 mg)] x 12 weeks in patients without NS5A resistant associated substitutions (RASs). 12 weeks duration recommended for patients without cirrhosis or compensated cirrhosis. In patients with NS5A RASs (G1a polymorphisms at amino acid positions 28A/G/T, 30D/E/H/G/K/L/R, 31F/M/V, or 93C/H/N/S) for elbasvir, elbasvir/grazoprevir + RBV x 16 weeks treatment duration can be considered as an alternative regimen (for pts w/o cirrosis or compensated cirrhosis).

5) Daily fixed-dose combination of paritaprevir (150 mg)/ritonavir (100 mg)/ombitasvir (25 mg)/dasabuvir (600 mg) [Vikira XR] plus weight-based RBV** x 12 wks (alternative in pts with no cirrhosis).

6) Daily Sovaldi [sofosbuvir (400 mg)] plus daily Olysio [simeprevir (150 mg)] x 12 weeks (no cirrhosis) or 24 weeks +/- weight-based RBV** (alternative in pts with compensated cirrhosis without Q80K substitution)

7) Daily Daklinza [daclatasvir* (60 mg)] plus daily Sovaldi [sofosbuvir (400 mg)] x 12 weeks (no cirrhosis) or x 24 weeks +/- RBV** (alternative in pts with compensated cirrhosis)

Treatment naive w/ genotype 1b

1) Daily fixed-dose combination Mavyret [glecaprevir (300mg)/pibrentasvir (120mg) x8 weeks (no cirrhosis) or x12 weeks (compensated cirrhosis).

2) Daily fixed-dose combination of Zepatier [elbasvir (50 mg)/grazoprevir (100 mg)] x 12 weeks in patients without cirrhosis or compensated cirrhosis.

3) Daily fixed-dose combination of Harvoni [ledipasvir (90 mg) + sofosbuvir (400 mg)] x12 weeks in pts without cirrhosis or compensate cirrhosis. For pts who are non-black, HIV negative, and HCV RNA vial load <6 million IU/mL treat for 8 weeks.

4) Daily fixed-dose combination of Epclusa [sofosbuvir (400 mg)/velpatasvir (100 mg)] x12 weeks in pts without cirrhosis or compensate cirrhosis

5) Daily fixed-dose combination of paritaprevir (150 mg)/ritonavir (100 mg)/ombitasvir (25 mg)/dasabuvir (600 mg) [Vikira XR] x 12 weeks. (alternattive in pts without cirrhosis or compensate cirrhosis).

6) Daily Sovaldi [sofosbuvir (400 mg)] plus daily Olysio [simeprevir (150 mg)] x 12 weeks (alternative in pts without cirrhosis)

7) Daily Daklinza [daclatasvir* (60 mg)] plus daily Sovaldi [sofosbuvir (400 mg)] x 12 weeks (alternative in pts with without cirrhosis)

**Weight based ribavirin (RBV) dosing: <75kg=1000 mg/d in two divided doses; >75kg=1200 mg/d in two divided doses.

*Daclastavir dose may need to be adjusted based on co-administered CYP3A4 inhibitors or inducers (e.g with ATV/r: use daclastavir 30mg/d; with EFV, NVP, ETR: use daclastavir 90mg/d)

See Table 17 (page 49) for anti-HCV and ARV drug-drug interactions

TABLE 52: Treatment of Hepatitis C:

(Amer Assoc for Study of Liver Diseases (AALSD) and Infectious Disease Society of America (IDSA) (http://www.hcvguidelines.org accessed 07/21/2017)

Treatment naive w/ genotype 2

1) Daily fixed-dose combination Mavyret [glecaprevir (300mg)/pibrentasvir (120mg) x8 weeks (no cirrhosis) or x12 weeks (compensated cirrhosis).

2) Daily fixed-dose combination of Epclusa [sofosbuvir (400 mg)/velpatasvir (100 mg)] x 12 wks for patients without cirrhosis and compensated cirrhosis.

Alternative: Sovaldi [sofosbuvir (400 mg)] daily plus Daklinza [daclatasvir* (60 mg)] daily x 12 wks (no cirrhosis) With compensated cirrhosis, extend treatment duration to 16-24 weeks.

Treatment naive w/ genotype 3

1) Daily fixed-dose combination Mavyret [glecaprevir (300mg)/pibrentasvir (120mg) x8 weeks (no cirrhosis) or x12 weeks (compensated cirrhosis).

2) Daily fixed-dose combination of Epclusa [sofosbuvir (400 mg)/velpatasvir (100 mg)] x 12 weeks for patients without cirrhosis and compensated cirrhosis.

Alternative: Daily Daklinza [daclatasvir* (60 mg)] plus Sovaldi [sofosbuvir (400 mg)] daily x 12 weeks (no cirrhosis) OR x 24 weeks +/- RBV** (compensated cirrhosis). In patients compensated cirrhosis, RAS testing for Y93H is recommended. Add weight-based RBV** to daclatasvir/sofosbuvir if Y93H is present.

Alternative: Daily fixed-dose combination Vosevi [sofosbuvir (400mg)/velpatasvir (100mg)/ voxilaprevir (100mg) (pts with compensated cirrhosis with Y93H mutation)

Treatment naive w/ genotype 4

1) Daily fixed-dose combination Epclusa [sofosbuvir (400 mg)/velpatasvir (100 mg)] x 12 weeks in patients without cirrhosis or compensated cirrhosis.

2) Daily fixed-dose combination Mavyret [glecaprevir (300mg)/pibrentasvir (120mg) x8 weeks (no cirrhosis) or x12 weeks (compensated cirrhosis).

3) Daily fixed-dose combination Harvoni [ledipasvir (90 mg)+ sofosbuvir (400 mg)] x 12 wks in pts without cirrhosis or compensated cirrhosis.

4) Daily fixed-dose combination Zepatier [elbasvir (50 mg)/grazoprevir (100 mg)] x 12 weeks in patients without cirrhosis or compensated cirrhosis.

Alternaive: Daily fixed-dose combination Technivie [paritaprevir (150mg)/ritonavir (100mg) x 12 weeks for pts without cirrhosis or compensated cirrhosis (add RBV in pts with compensated cirrhosis.

Treatment naive w/ genotype 5 or genotype 6

1) Daily fixed-dose combination Mavyret [glecaprevir (300mg)/pibrentasvir (120mg) x8 weeks (no cirrhosis) or x12 weeks (compensated cirrhosis).

2) Daily fixed-dose combination of Harvoni [ledipasvir (90 mg) + sofosbuvir (400 mg)] x 12 wks in pts without cirrhosis or compensate cirrhosis.

3) Daily fixed-dose combination of Epclusa [sofosbuvir (400 mg)/velpatasvir (100 mg)] x 12 wks in pts without cirrhosis or compensate cirrhosis.

HCV Treatment experienced: see www.hcvguidelines.org

**Weight based ribavirin (RBV) dosing: <75kg=1000 mg/d in two divided doses; >75kg=1200 mg/d in two divided doses.

*Daclastavir dose may need to be adjusted based on co-administered CYP3A4 inhibitors or inducers (e.g with ATV/r: use daclastavir 30mg/d; with EFV, NVP, ETR: use daclastavir 90mg/d)

See Table 17 (page 49) for anti-HCV an ARV drug-drug interactions

TABLE 53: Sexually Transmitted Disease*

(CDC 2015 STD guidelines http://www.cdc.gov/std/tg2015/)

Condition	Clinical Presentation/ Screening	Diagnosis
Urethritis/ Cervicitis	• Sx: Male-dysuria; urethral discharge; Female-cervical discharge+/- friable cervix • Many cases are asymptomatic • Etiologic agents: GC and non-gonococcal (C. trachomatis, M genitalium, Trichomonas and others) • Review of hx at follow-up visits, including contacts	N. gonorrhoeae + C. Trachomatis: NAAT first voided urine. Alternative: 1st voided urine for Gram, methylene blue, or gentian violet stain to detect gonococci (intracellular diplococci Inflammation (>2 WBC/oil immersion fie with neg GC stain is presumptive C. trachomatis.
Gonorrhea	• Dx: NAAT test-1st void urine and vaginal swabs (NAAT tests appropriate for rectal and pharyngeal swabs, though not FDA approved) • Sequela in females: PID, ectopic pregnancy and infertility. • Most common presentation: urethritis or cervicitis • Extra-genital sites of GC infection: oropharyngeal, rectal, conjunctival, and disseminated (DGI) • Review of Hx at follow-up visits, including contact with known other cases • Many infections are asymptomatic in men and women: consider urinary NAAT for GC & CT in sexually active men and women, including contacts with established cases. • Pharyngeal and anal testing in at risk patients	Gram stain or methylene blue and/or cul (or other specific test) of urethral or cerv swabs. Urine NAAT tests are valid for urethral infections, are most sensitive an usually more acceptable to patients. Limitation is lack of antibiotic sensitivitie Alternative agent: M. genitalium
Chlamydia	• Patient self-report Sx • Review of Hx at follow-up visits, including contacts • Most infections are asymptomatic • Consider as routine cervical test for sexually active women < 25 yrs. Consider routine NAAT urine test for GC & CT in sexually active women > 25 yrs and men • Consider repeat test annually, or more often with high risk	Culture is infrequently available. Alternatives are OFA, EIA, and NAAT on urethral and cervical specimens. Urine NAAT tests are sensitive and often preferred
Syphilis	• Patient self-report Sx • Contact with case • Screen at initial visit • Repeat screen annually	• Non-treponemal test (VDRL or RPR) plus treponemal test (FTA-ABS, TP-PA or EIA • Non-treponemal test (RPR, VDRL) titers reflect disease activity including respons treatment • Darkfield exam or OFA of lesion mater or exudates (primary syphilis)

† Screening interval depends upon community prevalence, outcome of previous tests, and risk

‡ Tetracycline, fluoroquinolones contraindicated in pregnancy

resumptive treatment of GC/CT for patients at risk (< 25 yrs, new sex partner, sex partner with oncurrent partners, or sex partner w/ STDs)

n persistent and recurrent non-GC urethritis, consider Mycoplasma genitalium that is implicated in 0% of non-GC cases. If initially treated with doxycycline: give azithromycin 1gm x1

 initially treated with azithromycin: give moxifloxacin 400 mg once daily x 7days

eterosexual men in a high T. vaginalis prevalence area: metronidazole 2g x1 or tinidazole 2 gm x1

rethral, endocervical, rectal, pharyngeal: Ceftriaxone 250 mg IM x 1 plus azithromycin 1gm po x 1

even if C. trachomatis is ruled out)

ote: 2015 changes in treatment recs are based on resistance reported to cefixime and increasing MICs o doxycycline. Treatment failure to cephalosporin should prompt culture and sensitivity testing.

lternative to azithromycin: Doxycycline 100 mg bid x 7 days. Alternative to ceftriaxone: cefixime 400mg 1

ephalosporin allergy: gemifloxacin 320 mg x1 PLUS azithromycin 2 gm (plus test-of-cure at 1 week) OR entamicin 240 mg IM x 1 PLUS azithromycin 2gm

Conjunctivitis: ceftriaxone 1gm IM plus azithromycin 1gm x1

Sex partners for past 60 days: Refer for evaluation and treatment

Test of cure testing recommended for pharyngeal GC

isseminated GC:

Dx: Culture or NAAT testing from multiple sites plus sensitivity testing.

Arthritis-Dermatitis: Ceftriaxone 1 gm/d IM or IV until improved for 24-48 h plus azithromycin 1gm po x , then ≥ 1 wk treatment with oral agents based on sensitivity tests: cefixime 400 mg qd or ciprofloxacin 00 mg bid or ofloxacin 400 mg bid or levofloxacin 500 mg qd. High rates of fluoroquinolone resistance eported nationally; check local resistance pattern

zithromycin** 1 gm po x 1 or
oxycycline‡** 100 mg po bid x 7 d

regnancy: Azithromycin 1gm po x 1

lternative: Amoxicillin 500 mg tid x 7 d or erythromycin regimen (above doses)

* Failure with doxycycline: Azithromycin 1 gm x 1. Failure with azithromycin: moxifloxacin 400 g/d x 7 d

Consider pharyngeal and anal testing in at risk patients

ee Table 54 (page 102): Management of Syphillis Co-Infection: Summary

Prophylaxis recommended for contact with syphilis: Benzathine Penicillin G 2.4 MU IM x 1 dose

(continued)

TABLE 53: Sexually Transmitted Disease* (cont.)

(CDC 2015 STD guidelines http://www.cdc.gov/std/tg2015/)

Condition	Identification / Screening	Diagnosis
Herpes simplex	• Recurrent genital ulcers • Most common cause of genital ulcer disease in the US and the world • Many infections are asymptomatic with viral shedding and transmission	• Patients with lesions suspected to herpes should be evaluated. • PCR is preferred test; culture, Tzanck test and IAFA are less sensitive • Serology for HSV-2 most sensitive test for HSV-2 infection, but not for Dx of herpes outbreak
Trichomonas	Malodorous yellow-green vaginal discharge	Wet mount or culture; NAAT is highly sensitive and detects 3-5 fold more cases compared to wet-mount microscopy
Bacterial Vaginosis	"Fishy smelling" vaginal discharge	3 of the following: • Clue cells (vaginal epithelial cells with adherent coccobacillus) • pH vaginal fluid > 4.5 • Fishy odor with 10% KOH • Thin white discharge on vaginal wall
Pelvic inflammatory disease	Diverse symptoms reflecting inflammation of the upper female genital tract with endometritis and salpingitis. Suspect with sexually active female with unexplained pelvic or lower abdominal pain. Physical exam shows cervical motion, uterine and/or adnexal tenderness.	• Oral temp >101° F • Mucopurulent cervical discharge • Vaginal fluid with abundant WBC • Increased ESR, CRP • Diagnosis of GC or CT

* CDC STD treatment guidelines updated by authors to reflect latest research data

Treatment			
	Acyclovir	Famciclovir	Valacyclovir
...V and no HIV			
...tial Episode	400 mg tid x 7-10 d	250 mg tid x 7-10 d	1 gm bid x 7-10 d
...isodic	400 mg tid x 5 d or 800 mg bid x 5 d or 800 mg tid x 2 d	125 mg bid x 5 d or 1000 mg bid x 1 d	500 mg bid x 3 d or 1 gm qd x 5 d
...ppression	400-800 mg tid	250 mg bid	500 mg or 1gm qd
...V and HIV			
...isodic	400 mg bid or tid x 5-10 d	500 mg bid x 7-10 d	1 gm bid x 5-10 d
...ppression	400-800 mg bid or tid	500 mg bid	500 mg bid

...tronidazole 2 gm 1X OR metronidazole 500 mg bid x 7 d
...irst regimen fails, metronidazole or tinidazole 2g once-daily x 7 days. Test susceptibility.

...tronidazole 500 mg bid x 7 d OR metronidazole gel 0.75% 5g intravaginal qd x 5 d OR
...damycin 2% cream 5g intravaginally qhs x 7 d
...ernative: Tinidazole 2g po qd x 2 d; tinidazole 1g po qd x 5 d; clindamycin 300 mg bid x 7 d;
...damycin ovules 100 mg intravaginally qhs x 3 d.

...ramuscular/Oral regimen
...triaxone 250 mg IM x 1 plus doxycycline 100 mg bid x 14 d +/- metronidazole 500 mg po bid x
...d
...oxitin 2 gm x 1 plus probenicid 1 gm po x 1 plus doxycycline 100 mg bid x 14 d +/-
...tronidazole 500 mg po x 14 d
...er 3rd generation cephalosporin plus doxycycline 100 mg bid x 14 d +/- metronidazole 500 mg
...bid x 14 d

...enteral: Cefoxitin 2 gm IV q6h OR cefotetan 2gm IV q12h
...LUS doxycycline 100 mg po or IV q12h until improved,
...HEN doxycycline 100 mg bid po to complete 14 d
...enteral alternative: Ampicillin/sulbactam 3gm IV q6h
...LUS doxycycline IV or PO 100 mg q12h to complete 14 d course

TABLE 54: Management of Syphilis Co-Infection: Summary*

Form	Treatment	LP†
Primary and secondary syphilis	• Initial: Benzathine penicillin G 2.4 mil units IM x 1 • Penicillin allergy****: doxycycline 100 mg po bid x 14 d or ceftriaxone 1 gm qd IV or IM x 8-10 d or azithromycin*** 2 gm po x 1 • Re-treatment: Benzathine penicillin G 2.4 mil units IM x 3 (weekly)	• Neuro SX • Titer increases 4-fol • SX persist or recur
Early latent (< 1 year)	• Initial: Benzathine penicillin G 2.4 mil units IM x 1 • Penicillin allergy****: doxycycline 100 mg po bid x 14 d or ceftriaxone 1 gm qd IV or IM x 8-10 d or azithromycin*** 2 gm po x 1 • Re-treatment: Benzathine penicillin G 2.4 mil units IM x 3 (weekly)	• Neuro SX • SX persist or recur
Late latent (> 1 year or unknown duration)	• Benzathine penicillin G 2.4 mil units IM weekly for 3 weeks • Penicillin allergy****: doxycycline 100 mg po bid x 28 days‡	• All HIV-infected patients
Late syphilis (tertiary, not neurosyphilis)	• Benzathine penicillin G 2.4 mil units IM weekly for 3 weeks • Penicillin allergy****: doxycycline 100 mg po bid x 28 days‡	• All patients
Neurosyphilis** (or ocular, otic syphilis)	• Aq penicillin G, 18-24 mil units/d x 10-14 d administered as 3-4 million units IV q4h • Alternative: Procaine penicillin 2.4 million units IM qd + probenecid 500 mg po qid x 10-14 d • Penicillin allergy: Skin testing to confirm allergy and/or PCN desensitization with consultant expertise, then treat with penicillin (preferred). If PCN desensitization is not feasible, ceftriaxone 2 gm qd IV or IM x 10-14 d (risk of cross-reaction is low but not zero)	• Required

* CDC 2015 STD treatment guidelines and 2015 OI guidelines
† Some experts recommend CSF examinations of all syphilis-H IV co-infected patients before treatment, regardless of stage, and modification of treatment accordingly. Consultation with an expert may be appropriate.
‡ Alteratives to penicillin have not been sufficiently evaluated in HIV infected persons and cannot be considered first-line therapy. If required, there needs to be close clinical monitoring. If adherence cannot be assured, desensitization and treatment with penicillin is recommended.
**CSF VDRL is very specific bu not very sensitive. It is the only approved CSF syphilis test. Consider CNS syphilis if other conditions ruled out and CSF WBC >20. Note that CSF FTA-abs is not specific but may help rule out neurosyphilis (Harding AS, Sex Trans Dis 2012; 39: 291)
***High rates of azithromycin resistance in MSM. Not recommended in MSM and pregnant pts.
****PCN desensitization and Benzathine PCN recommended in non-adherent or if follow-up cannot be ensured.

Follow-up VDRL/RPR	Expectation VDRL/RPR	Indications to Re-treat
3, 6, 9, 12, and 24 mos	4-fold decrease at 6-12 mos	• Titer increases four-fold • Titer fails to decrease four-fold at 6-12 mos • Symptoms persist or recur • Jarish-Herxheimer reaction (fever, h/a, myalgia) can occur in the first 24hrs.
3, 6, 12, 18, and 24 mos	4-fold decrease at 12-24 mos	• Titer increases four-fold • Titer of > 1:32 fails to decrease four-fold at 12-24 mos • Develops signs or sx of syphilis • Jarish-Herxheimer reaction (fever, h/a, myalgia) can occur in the first 24hrs.
3, 6, 12, 18, and 24 mos	4-fold decrease at 6-12 mos (lower initial titers may remain unchanged)	• Titer fails to decrease four-fold at 12-24 mos • Increase titer by four-fold at any time after 3 mos
6 and 12 mos	• As above • Granulomatous lesions should heal	• As above • Documentation of T. pallidum or other histologic features of late syphilis
Every 6 mos until CSF normal	CSF WBC decrease at 6 mos and CSF normal at 24 mos	• CSF WBC fails to decrease at 6 mos or CSF VDRL is still positive • Persisting signs and symptoms • Avoid probenecid with history of severe sulfonamide allergy • Consider benzathine PCN 2.4 MU weekly x 3 weeks after completion of IV PCN. • Jarish-Herxheimer reaction (fever, h/a, myalgia) can occur in the first 24hrs.

TABLE 55: Occupational Post·Exposure Prophylaxis (PEP) (MMWR 2015; 63: 1245 and Kuhar et al. USPHS Guidelines, Infect Control Hosp Epidemiol 2013; 34 (9): 875)

Exposure
Percutaneous injury with sharp object or exposure to mucous membranes or nonintact skin (skin that is abraded, chapped or with dermatitis)

Risk
- US data from occupational HIV transmissions for 1985 to 2013: 58 confirmed and 150 possible cases. There was only one confirmed case from 2000-2012 (Joyce MP MMWR 2015; 63: 1245)
- Prospective studies of transmission risk in the pre-HAART era showed 1) 20/6135 (0.33%) following percutaneous exposure; 2) 1/1143 (0.09%) following mucous membrane exposure; and 3) 0/2712 intact skin exposures (Henderson DK. Ann Intern Med 1990; 113: 740). More recent CDC guidance still quote a risk of 0.3% for occupationally-acquired HIV with a needlestick injury from an HIV infected source despite more recent low number of reported events with only one confirmed case in U.S. (Henderson DK. JAMA 2012; 307:75)

Management
Exposed site: Immediate cleansing of exposed site-1) skin: soap and water; 2) puncture wounds: alcohol-based hand wipes; 3) mucosal surface: flush with water; 4) eyes: saline or water irrigation
- Establish HIV status of source by history or rapid HIV test (with consent)
- Counseling HCW: 1) Risk (as summarized above); 2) risk for other bloodborne pathogens-HBV and HCV; 3) abstain or safe sex until serologic testing completed and negative
- HIV testing: 4th generation test that combines HIV p24 antigen-HIV antibody (preferred). Test at baseline, 6 weeks, 3 months, and 6 months.
- Medical treatment within 72 hours.(effectiveness presumably declines with each hour of delay (CDC MMWR 2005; 54 (RR2:1-20):

ART Regimens: see Table 57 (page 105)

Need for Expert Consultations (Call: PEPline 888-448-4911)
- 1) Delayed exposure report (>72 hrs); 2) unknown source; 3) known or suspected pregnancy; 4) breast feeding exposed person; 5) suspected HIV resistance in exposed person; 6) toxicity to PEP regimen; 7) serious medical condition in infected source.

TABLE 56: Non-Occupational Post·Exposure Prophylaxis (nPEP) (CDC and DHHS updated 2016 Guidelines for ARV nPEP after sexual, IVDU, or other nonoccupational Exposure to HIV)

Criteria for high risk exposure: Isolated exposure to source with known HIV infection or high risk (MSM, IVDU, sex worker) within 72 hours can be evaluated for nPEP
Exposed site: Mucous membrane (vagina, rectum, mouth, eye), non intact skin or percutaneous
Exposure to: Blood or bloody fluid, vaginal or rectal secretions, or breast milk

Risk-Single exposure from infected source (CDC MMWR 2005 RR02; 54; Varghese B. Sex Transm Dis 2002; 29:37; http://www.cdc.gov/hiv/policies/law/risk.html accessed 7/17)
1) Parenteral-63/10,000: Needle-sharing IVDU; 23/10,000: percutaneous needle stick
2) Sexual-138/10,000: receptive anal intercourse; 8/10,000: receptive vaginal intercourse;   11/10,000: insertive anal intercourse; 4:10,000: insertive vaginal intercourse; 0.5-1/10,000: Receptive oral intercourse.
3) Other-biting, spiting, throwing body fluids (semen, saliva), sharing sex toys: negligible risk

Timing: Medical treatment within 72 hours

ART Regimens: see Table 57, page 105). Treatment not recommended for patients presenting >72 hours after exposure or if risk of HIV acquisition is negligible.

Laboratory testing for source and exposed person: See Table 58

Post-exposure monitoring:
• HIV test of exposed person:

4th generation test with HIV p24 Ag and HIV Ab (preferred for early detection): baseline, 4-6 weeks, and 3 months or with any symptoms suggesting acute HIV infection. P24 Ag should be detected at about 8-10 days. HIV RNA will be detected earlier. Report any seroconversion to CDC at 1-800-893-0485

TABLE 57: PEP and nPEP Recommended Regimens

	Regimen (4 week duration)
Preferred	RAL 400 mg bid OR DTG* 50 mg qd plus TDF/FTC 300/200 mg qd
Alternative	DRV/r 800/100 mg qd plus TDF/FTC 300/200 mg qd
For Pts with CrCL <60ml/min	Preferred: RAL 400 mg bid OR DTG* 50 mg qd plus AZT + 3TC Alternative: DRV/r 800/100 mg qd plus AZT + 3TC

* Dolutegravir-based regimen recommended in the nPEP guidelines, but also recommended by authors for occupational PEP. Consult expert if source patient known to harbor drug-resistant HIV

TABLE 58: nPEP (and PEP) Lab Monitoring

	Source	Exposed Patient			
Test	Baseline	Baseline	Wk 4-6	3 months	6 months
Rapid combined Ag/Ab (4th Gen)	+	+	+	+	recheck if new HCV infection*
HIV viral load/ HIV genotypic resistance	+	check at first visit where determined to be HIV+			
STDs (GC, chlamydia, syphilis)	+	+	If symptomatic	-	If +syphylis and treated
HCV Ab	+	+	-	-	If source+
HBsAg, HBsAb, HB core Ab	+	+	-	-	If source+ and pt not immune
Serum Cr; LFTs	-	If Rx TDF/FTC plus [DTG or RAL]		-	-
Pregnancy Test	-	+	+	-	-

* Delayed HIV seroconversion observed in patients who simultaneously acquire HIV and HCV infection

Resources for PEP

- PEPline:
  http://nccc.ucsf.edu/
  Telephone: 1-888-448-4911--

- Hepatitis Hotline:
  Telephone: 1-888-443-7232

- Report Occupational Exposure with Transmission: CDC guidance
  Telephone: 1-800-893-0485 or 404-639-2050

- HIV Pregnancy registry:
  http://www.apregistry.com/
  Telephone: 1-800-258-4263
  Email: registry@nc.crl.com

- HIV/AIDS Treatment Information Service:
  http://aidsinfo.nih.gov/

TABLE 59: Pre-Exposure Prophylaxis (PrEP) (2017 CDC Recommendations)

(https://www.cdc.gov/hiv/pdf/risk/prep/cdc-hiv-prep-guidelines-2017.pdf) Clinician Supplement (https://www.cdc.gov/hiv/pdf/risk/prep/cdc-hiv-prep-provider-supplement-2017.pdf)

Indications
Indications: MSM at substantial risk of HIV acquisition
1) Adult male; 2) no acute or chronic HIV infection; 3) male sex partner in past 6 months; 4) not in a monogamous relationship with recently tested HIV negative man
        PLUS
1) Anal sex without condoms in past 6 months; 2) any sexually transmitted infection diagnosed or reported in past 6 months;
Indications: Heterosexual men and women
1) Adult; 2) no acute or chronic HIV infection; 3) any heterosexual sex in past 6 months;4) not in monogamous relationship with recently tested HIV negative partner
        AND at least one of the following:
1) Infrequent use of condoms with one or more partners with unknown HIV status who are at "substantial HIV risk" (IDU or bisexual male); 2) in ongoing sexual relationship with HIV positive partner. 3)any bacterial sexually transmitted infection diagnosed or reported in past 6 months. 4)Man who has sex with men and women

Indications: Injection drug users (IDUs)
1) Adult; 2) no acute or chronic HIV infection; 3) injection of drugs not physician prescribed in past 6 months
        PLUS one of the following:
1) Sharing injection or drug preparation equipment in past 6 months; 2) been in a methadone, buprenorphine or suboxone treatment program in past 6 months; OR 3) risk of sexual transmission of HIV (see above)

Recommended oral PrEP medications
Regimen: TDF/FTC 300/200 mg po once daily. Note: TAF/FTC not recommended
Clinically eligible: 1)Documented negative HIV test prior to prescribing. 2)No signs of acute HIV 3)Normal renal function 4)Documented HBV infection/vaccination status
Time to Protection: Estimated at 7 days for rectal sex and 20 days for vaginal sex (based on tissue concentrations)
Monitoring Every 3 months: 1) HIV test; 2) refills for no more than 3 months; 3) pregnancy test for conception vulnerable q 3 months; 4) support for adherence and risk prevention;5) assess side effects, adherence, risk behavior 6)Conduct STI testing for sexually active persons with signs/sx of infection, and asymptomatic MSM
Monitoring Every 6 months: 1) declining CrCL but > 60ml/min -- consult nephrologist; 2) test for sexually transmitted disease if sexually active even if asymptomatic -- syphilis, gonorrhea, Chlamydia trachomatis.
Drug interactions: TDF: possible increases of either TDF or interacting drug: acyclovir, valacyclovir, cidofovir, ganciclovir, valganciclovir; drugs that reduce renal function, including aminoglycoside, high-dose or multiple NSAIDs.
FTC: no data with drugs listed above, but interaction unlikely

Risk reduction counseling
Establish trust and communication
Support risk reduction efforts
Monitor behavioral adherence in non-judgmental manner

"ADDITIONAL INFORMATION

"As needed Coitally Dependent PrEP"
The IPERGAY trial tested the efficacy of TDF/FTC given prophylactically prior and after the time of anticipated sex in a high risk population of seronegative MSM who had frequent sex. The TDF/FTC vs. placebo controlled trial showed that prophylaxis using the regimen described below was 86% effective (p<0.01) in preventing HIV transmission

The regimen: 2 TDF/FTC (Truvada) pills at 2-24 hrs before sex (or one pill if the last dose was 1-6 days previously) and 2 doses 24 and 48 hrs after the pre-sex dose. Because of the high frequency of sex and pill taking in the study population, it is not known if alternatives a few hours/days before sex will work. Consequently, the FDA and CDC do not yet recommend non-daily TDF/FTC for PReP

Note: TAF/FTC not yet recommended. Ongoing clinical trials.

"Transition PrEP" or "Bridge PrEP":
This method employs PrEP in the standard TDF/FTC regimen (1 pill/day) for discordant couples in which the uninfected partner uses PrEP regimen during the period required by the infected partner to achieve viral suppression with ART.

The CDC issued a statement 2/24/15 urging people at "substantial risk" for HIV infection to take steps to reduce this risk by encouraging PrEP by MSM, heterosexual men and women and IDUs (CDC statement 2/24/15
http://cdc.gov/nchhstp/newsroom/2015/IPERGAY-2015-Media-Statement.html

US preventative services task force: Nov 2018 issued a draft statement on usage of PrEP: "The USPSTF recommends that clinicians offer pre-exposure prophylaxis (PrEP) with effective antiretroviral therapy to persons who are at high risk of HIV acquisition.", Grade A. The found no accurate tools to assess risk of HIV acquision. USPTF recommends PrEP be considered in:
1.MSM with one of the following: a)serdiscordant sex partner; recent STI; inconsistent condom usage during receptive or insertive anal sex
2.Heterosexual men and women who are sexually active and have one of the following: a)serodiscordant couple b)inconsistent condom usage with partner whose HIV status is unknown or is at high risk c)recent STI with syphilis or gonorrhea
3. Persons that inject drug that share injection equpiment, or have sexual risk above
https://www.uspreventiveservicestaskforce.org/Page/Document/draft-recommendation-statement/prevention-of-human-immunodeficiency-virus-hiv-infection-pre-exposure-prophylaxis

TABLE 60: Dosing of antimicrobial agents for Patients with Chronic Kidney Disease (CKD) or End-Stage Renal Disease (ESRD).

Adapted from Clinical Practice Guideline for the Management of Chronic Kidney Disease in Patients Infected with HIV: 2014 HIVMA/IDSA CID 2014.

Drug, dosing category	Dosage
Abacavir	
No dose adjustment with CKD or ESRD	600 mg po q24h or 300 mg po q12h
Acyclovir	
Cr CL > 50 mL/min	Usual dosage (high dose for zoster): 200–800 mg po 3-5 times per day; 5–10 mg per kg of ideal body weight IV q8h
Cr CL 25-50 mL/min	200-800 mg po 3-5 times per day; 5-10 mg/kg IV q12h
Cr CL 10-24 mL/min	200-800 mg po q8h; 5-10 mg/kg IV q24h
Cr CL < 10 mL/min	200-800 mg q12h; 2.5–5 mg per kg of ideal body weight IV q24h
Cr CL < 10 mL/min receiving hemodialysis	2.5–5 mg per kg of ideal body weight IV q24h. On days of HD, dose post-HD.
Amikacin	
Cr CL > 60 mL/min	Mycobacterial Infections: 15 mg/kg/d IV or 25 mg/kg TIW
Cr CL < 60 mL/min	Adjust dose based on serum concentrations. Target peak 35–45 mcg/mL and trough <4 mcg/mL.
Amphotericin B deoxycholate	
Cr CL > 50 mL/min	Usual dosage: 0.7-1.0 mg/kg iv q24h
Dosage for patients with CKD	No dose adjustment (but consider lipid amphotericin formulations, azoles, or echinocandins)
Amphotericin B liposomal	
Cr CL > 50 mL/min	Usual dosage: 4.0–6.0 mg per kg of actual body weight iv q24h
Dosage for patients with CKD or ESRD	No dose adjustment
Atazanavir	
No dose adjustment with CKD or ESRD	ATV/r 300/100 mg once-daily or ATV 400 mg once-daily
Receiving hemodialysis	Avoid unboosted ATV. Avoid boosted ATV in treatment-experienced patients with PI resistant mutations.
Azithromycin	
No dose adjustment with CKD or ESRD	
Bictegravir/Tenofovir alafenamide/emtricitabine	
Cr CL > 30 mL/min Cr CL < 30 mL/min	BIC/TAF/FTC 50mg/25mg/200mg tab once daily Avoid co-formulation with CrCL < 30 mL/min
Ceftriaxone	
No dose adjustment with CKD or ESRD	1-2 gm IM or IV once-daily; GC: 250 mg IM x 1;Meningitis: 2gm IV q12h
Cidofovir	
Cr CL > 55 mL/min and a urine protein < 100 mg/dL	Usual dosage: 5 mg per/kg IV q week x 2 weeks, then every other week (with probenecid and hydration)
Increase in serum creatinine level to 0.3–0.4 above baseline	3 mg per kg of body weight iv every other week (with probenecid and hydration)
Increase in serum creatinine level to ≥ 0.5 above baseline or development of grade 3+ proteinuria	Discontinue

TABLE 60: Dosing of antimicrobial agents for Patients with Chronic Kidney Disease (CKD) or End-Stage Renal Disease (ESRD).

Drug, dosing category	Dosage
Cidofovir (cont.)	
Baseline serum creatinine level >1.5, creatinine clearance ≤ 55 mL/min, or grade ≥ 2+ proteinuria	Not recommended
Ciprofloxacin	
Cr CL > 50 mL/min	Usual dosage: 500-750 mg po q12h OR 400 IV q8h-12h
Cr CL 30–50 mL/min	500-750 mg q12h OR 400 IV q12h
Cr CL < 30 mL/min	250–500 mg q18-24h OR 400 IV q24h
Receiving hemodialysis	250–500 mg q24h OR 200-400 IV q24h (days of HD dose post-HD)
Clarithromycin	
Cr CL > 30 mL/min	Usual dosage: 500 mg po q12h With ATV co-administration, reduce clarithromycin dose by 50%. With other PI co-administration, dose reduction by 50% with CrCL 30-60 mL/min.
Cr CL < 30 mL/min	Reduce dose by one half if creatinine clearance <30 mL/min. With PI co-administration, 75% reduction with CrCL <30 mL/min
Daclatasvir	
No dose adjustment with CKD or ESRD	60 mg po once-daily (in combination with sofosbuvir. See sofosbuvir for dosing with CrCL < 30 ml/min).
Dapsone	
No dose adjustment with CKD or ESRD	PCP prophylaxis: 100 mg once-daily PCP treatment (mild to moderate disease): 100 mg once-daily (in combination with trimethoprim)
DRV/r/TAF/FTC	**Not recommended if CrCL <30ml/min**
Darunavir	
No dose adjustment with CKD or ESRD	DRV/r 800/100 mg once-daily or DRV/r 600/100 mg twice-daily
Didanosine EC		
Cr CL ≥ 60 mL/min	Body weight >60 kg	400 mg q24h
Cr CL 30–59 mL/min		200 mg q24h
Cr CL 10–29 mL/min		125 mg q24h
Cr CL < 10 mL/min		125 mg q24h
Receiving HD or PD		125 mg q24h
Cr CL ≤ 60 mL/min	Body weight <60 kg	250 mg q24h
Cr CL 30–59 mL/min		125 mg q24h
Cr CL 10–29 mL/min		125 mg q24h
Cr CL < 10 mL/min		75 mg (pediatric powder for suspension) q24h
Receiving HD or PD		75 mg (pediatric powder for suspension) q24h
DTG/ABC/3TC	**Co-formulation not recommended with CrCL <50 ml/min**
Dolutegravir	
Cr CL > 30 ml/min	50 mg once-daily (ARV- or INSTI-naïve patients) 50 mg twice-daily (INSTI-experienced with certain INSTI mutations)

TABLE 60: Dosing of antimicrobial agents for Patients with Chronic Kidney Disease (CKD) or End-Stage Renal Disease (ESRD).

Drug, dosing category	Dosage
Dolutegravir (cont.)	
Cr CL < 30 ml/min	Use usual dose (above). DTG concentrations decreased by 40%. Clinical significance unknown, but INSTI-experienced patients with INSTI mutations may be at increased risk for virologic breakthrough.
Doravirine	No dose adjustment with CKD; <15ml/min: no data. Usual dose likely
Doravirine/TDF/FTC	CrCL >50ml/min: SD; not recommended with CrCL <50ml/min
Doxycycline	
No dose adjustment with CKD or ESRD	100 mg po twice-daily.
Efavirenz	
No dose adjustment with CKD or ESRD	600 mg po qhs
Elbasvir- Grazoprevir	
No dose adjustment with CKD	Usual dose: Elbasvir 50mg- Grazoprevir 100mg po once daily
Elvitegravir	
No dose adjustment with CKD when combined with boosted PI	EVG 85 mg once-daily + ATV/r 300/100 mg once-daily EVG 150 mg once-daily + DRV/r 600/100 mg twice-daily
Cr CL ≥ 70 mL/min	EVG/COBI/TDF/FTC 150/150/300/200 mg (Stribild) 1 tablet po q24h. D/C if Cr CL < 50 ml/min.
Cr CL ≥ 30 mL/min	EVG/COBI/TAF/FTC 150/150/10/200 mg (Genvoya) 1 tablet po q24h. D/C if Cr CL < 30 ml/min.
Emtricitabine	
Cr CL ≥ 50 mL/min	200 mg po q24h
Cr CL 30–49 mL/min	200 mg po q48h
Cr CL 15–29 mL/min	200 mg po q 3 days
Cr CL < 15 mL/min	200 mg po q 4 days
Receiving hemodialysis	200 mg po q 4 days
Receiving peritoneal dialysis	No data. Dose reduction needed
Enfuvirtide	
No dose adjustment with CKD or ESRD	90 mg subcutaneous twice-daily
Entecavir	
Cr CL ≥ 50 mL/min	0.5 mg q24h (HBV treatment-naïve); 1 mg q24h (3TC-refractory HBV or with decompensated liver disease)
Cr CL 30-49 mL/min	0.25 mg q24h (HBV treatment-naïve); 0.5 mg q24h (3TC-refractory HBV or with decompensated liver disease)
Cr CL 10-29 mL/min	0.15 mg q24h (HBV treatment-naïve); 0.3 mg q24h (3TC-refractory HBV or with decompensated liver disease)
Cr CL < 10 mL/min; HD or PD	0.05 mg q24h or 0.5 mg q7d (HBV treatment-naïve); 0.1 mg q24h or 1 mg q7d (3TC-refractory HBV or with decompensated liver disease)
Ethambutol	
Cr CL > 50 mL/min	Usual dosage: 15–25 mg per kg of body weight po q24h
Cr CL 10–50 mL/min	15–25 mg per kg of body weight po q24–36h

TABLE 60: Dosing of antimicrobial agents for Patients with Chronic Kidney Disease (CKD) or End-Stage Renal Disease (ESRD).

Drug, dosing category		Dosage
Ethambutol (cont.)		
Cr CL < 10 mL/min		15–25 mg per kg of body weight po q48h
Etravirine		
No dose adjustment with CKD or ESRD		200 mg po twice-daily
Famciclovir		
Cr CL >60 mL/min Cr CL 40-59 mL/min		Usual dosage: 500 mg po q12h (HSV); 500 q8h (VZV) 500 mg q12h (HSV); 500 mg q12h (VZV)
Cr CL 20–39 mL/min		500 mg q24h
Cr CL < 20 mL/min		250 mg q24h
Receiving hemodialysis		250 mg after each dialysis
Fluconazole		
Cr CL > 50 mL/min		Usual dosage: 200-1200 mg po q24h
Cr CL = or < 50 mL/min		1/2 dose
Receiving hemodialysis		Full dose after dialysis
Flucytosine Monitor concentrations: target 30-80 mcg/mL (2hr post dose)		
Cr CL > 40 mL/min		Usual dosage: 25mg/kg q6h
Cr CL 20-40 mL/min		25 mg/kg q12h
Cr CL 10-20 mL/min		25 mg/kg q24h
Cr CL < 10 mL/min		25 mg/kg q48h
Fosamprenavir		
No dose adjustment with CKD or ESRD		FPV/r 1400/100 mg once-daily or FPV/r 700/100 mg twice-daily
Foscarnet		
CrCl (mL/min/kg)	CMV Induction Treatment	CMV Maintenance Treatment
>1.4	90mg/kg q12h	90 mg/kg q24h
1.0-1.4	70 mg/kg q12h	70 mg/kg q24h
0.8-1.0	50 mg/kg q12h	50 mg/kg q24h
0.6-0.8	80 mg/kg q24h	80 mg/kg q48h
0.5-0.6	60 mg/kg q24h	60 mg/kg q48h
0.4-0.5	50 mg/kg q24h	50 mg/kg q48h
<0.4	Not recommended	Not recommended
Ganciclovir		
Usual dosage		5mg/kg q12h (induction [I]); 5mg/kg q24h(maintenance [M])
50-69 mL/min		2.5 mg/kg q12h (I); 2.5 mg/kg q24h (M)
25-49 mL/min		2.5 mg/kg q24h (I); 1.25 mg/kg q24h (M)
10-24 mL/min		1.25 mg/kg q24h (I); 0.625 mg/kg q24h (M)
< 10 mL/min; HD		1.25 mg/kg TIW (I) post-HD; 0.625 mg/kg TIW (M) post-HD

TABLE 60: Dosing of antimicrobial agents for Patients with Chronic Kidney Disease (CKD) or End-Stage Renal Disease (ESRD).

Drug, dosing category	Dosage	
Glecaprevir-Pibrentasvir		
No dose adjustment with CKD or ESRD	Usual dose: Glecaprevir 300mg-Pibrentasvir 120 po mg once daily.	
Ibalizumab-uiyk	No data. Usual dose likely	
Indinavir		
No dose adjustment with CKD or ESRD	IDV/r 800/100 mg po twice-daily	
Isoniazid		
Cr CL > 10 mL/min	Usual dosage: 300 mg po q24h	
Cr CL < 10 mL/min	300 mg q24h (on days of HD, dose post-HD); consider dose adjustment in slow acetylators.	
Itraconazole		
No dose adjustment with CKD or ESRD	Candida esophagitis: 200 mg liquid once-daily Coccidioidomycosis: 200 mg twice-daily Target peak (2hr post-dose): > 1 mcg/mL	
Lamivudine		
Cr CL > 50 mL/min	300 mg po q 24h or 150 mg po q12h	
Cr CL 30–49 mL/min	150 mg po q 24h	
Cr CL 15–29 mL/min	150 mg po first dose, then 100 mg po q 24h	
Cr CL 5–14 mL/min	150 mg po first dose, then 50 mg* po q24h.	*To avoid using the liquid formulation and because of the favorable safety profile, the authors use lowest available tablet dose of 100 mg (lamivudine HB) or 150 mg (lamivudine) daily
Cr CL < 5mL/min, hemodialysis, or peritoneal dialysis	50 mg po first dose, then 25 mg* po q24h.	
Levofloxacin		
Cr CL > 50 mL/min	Usual dosage: 500–750 mg IV or po q24h	
Cr CL 20-49 mL/min	500mg loading dose, then 250 mg q24h	
Cr CL 10-19 mL/min	500mg loading dose, then 250 mg q48h	
Receiving hemodialysis or PD	750-500 mg loading dose, then 250-500 mg q48h (dose post-HD on days of dialysis)	
Lopinavir/ritonavir		
No dose adjustment with CKD or ESRD	400 mg/100 mg po twice-daily. OR 800 mg/200 mg po once-daily	
Receiving hemodialysis	LPV trough lower in HD, use with caution in patients with PI resistant mutations.	
Maraviroc		
Cr CL > 30 mL/min	300 mg po twice-daily	
Cr CL < 30 mL/min	300 mg po twice-daily Reduce dose to 150 mg po twice-daily if orthostatic hypotension occurs. Avoid MVC with CYP3A4 inhibitor (e.g. macrolides, azoles, protease inhibitors).	

TABLE 60: Dosing of antimicrobial agents for Patients with Chronic Kidney Disease (CKD) or End-Stage Renal Disease (ESRD).

Drug, dosing category	Dosage
Metronidazole	
No dose adjustment with CKD or ESRD	250-500 mg po q8h C. difficile: 500 po q8h x 10-14 days BV or Trichomonas: 500 mg po q12h x 7 days
Moxifloxacin	
No dose adjustment with CKD or ESRD	400 mg po or IV once-daily
Nelfinavir	
No dose adjustment with CKD or ESRD	1250 mg po twice-daily or 750 mg q8h
Nevirapine	
No dose adjustment with CKD or ESRD	Usual dose: 200 mg po twice-daily (after 2 weeks of 200 mg po once-daily)
ESDR on HD	Give additional 200 mg post-HD
Nitazoxanide	
No dose adjustment with CKD or ESRD	Cryptosporidiosis: 0.5-1.0 gm po twice-daily (in combination with ART)
Paritaprevir-Ritonavir- Ombitasvir- Dasabuvir	
No dose adjustment with CKD or ESRD	Usual dose: Paritaprevir 150mg-ritonavir 100mg- ombitasvir 25mg- dasabuvir 600mg (XR tablet) po once daily.
Paromomycin	
No dose adjustment with CKD or ESRD	Cryptosporidiosis: 500 mg po q6h (in combination with ART)
Penicillin G	
Cr CL > 50 mL/min	Streptococcal endocarditis, neurosyphilis or ocular syphilis: 3–4 MU IV q4h OR 18–24 MU continuous IV infusion daily
Cr CL 10-50 mL/min	2–3 MU IV q4h OR 12–18 MU continuous IV infusion daily.
Cr CL < 10 mL/min	2 MU IV q4–6h OR 8–12 MU continuous IV infusion daily.
Receiving HD or PD	2 MU IV q6h OR 8 MU continuous IV infusion daily.
Pentamidine	
Cr CL > 50 mL/min	Usual dosage: 4.0 mg per kg of body weight IV q24h
Cr CL 10–50 mL/min	3.0 mg per kg of body weight IV q24h (use with caution)
Cr CL < 10 mL/min	4.0 mg per kg of body weight iv q-48h
Posaconazole	
Cr CL > 50 mL/min	Esophageal candidiasis (refractory to fluconazole and itraconazole): 400 mg po q12h Invasive fungal infections: 300 mg IV q12h x 2 (load), then 300 mg IV once-daily, then transition to oral posaconazole once clinically stable (400 mg po twice-daily; up to 1200 mg/day based on clinical response and trough concentrations). Target trough for invasive infections > 1.25 mcg/mL
Cr CL < 50 mL/min	Usual oral posaconazole dose Large pharmacokinetic variability with Cr CL < 20 mL/min. Use with close monitoring. Target trough for invasive infections > 1.25 mcg/mL Avoid IV posaconazole because of potential toxicity due to accumulation of sulfobutylether-cyclodexrin (SBECD vehicle of IV product). Based on observational study with IV voriconazole, this appears to be not a genuine concern.

TABLE 60: Dosing of antimicrobial agents for Patients with Chronic Kidney Disease (CKD) or End-Stage Renal Disease (ESRD).

Drug, dosing category	Dosage
Pyrazinamide	
Cr CL > 10 mL/min	Usual dosage: 20–25 mg/kg (max 2 gm) po q24h
Cr CL < 10 mL/min	50% of usual dose
Receiving hemodialysis	Usual dose post-HD
Pyrimethamine	
No dose adjustment with CKD or ESRD	Toxoplasmosis treatment: 200 mg x 1, then 50 mg (<60 kg) or 75 mg (> 60 kg) po once-daily (in combination sulfadiazine or clindamycin)
Raltegravir	
No dose adjustment with CKD or ESRD	400 mg po twice-daily
Ribavirin	
Cr CL > 50 mL/min	Usual dosage: 800-1200 mg/day po in two divided doses.
Cr CL 30-50 mL/min	Alternate 200 mg and 400 mg every other day.
Cr CL < 30 mL/min	200 mg po qd
Cr CL < 10 mL/min on HD	200mg/d (limited data w/ high dropout rates).Avoid if possible
Rifabutin	
Cr CL > 30 mL/min	Usual dosage: 300 mg po q24h (dose adjustment needed with PI/r or PI/c co-administration)
Cr CL < 30 mL/min	Consider 50% dose reduction
Rifampin	
Cr CL > 50 mL/min	Usual dosage: 600 mg po q24h
Cr CL 10–50 mL/min	100% of full dose
Cr CL < 10 mL/min	50%–100% of full dose
Receiving hemodialysis	50%–100% of full dose; no supplement
Receiving peritoneal dialysis	50%–100% of full dose; extra 50%–100% of full dose after receipt of peritoneal dialysis. TDM recommended
Rilpivirine	
No dose adjustment with CKD or ESRD	RPV 25 mg po once-daily
CrCL ≥ 30 mL/min	RPV/TAF/FTC 25/25/200 mg tablet once-daily with food; If CrCL < 30 ml/min avoid RPV/TAF/FTC; If CrCL < 50 ml/min avoid RPV/TDF/FTC
Saquinavir	
No dose adjustment with CKD or ESRD	SQV/r 1000/100 mg po twice-daily
Simepravir	
No dose adjustment with CKD or ESRD	150 mg po once-daily (in combination with sofosbuvir). See sofosbuvir for CrCL <30 ml/min.
Sofosbuvir	
Cr CL > 30 ml/min	Usual dose: Sofosbuvir 400mg po once-daily (in combination with another HCV agent).
Cr CL < 30 ml/min	Dose not established. Significant increase in sofosbuvir metabolite (up to 20-fold). Clinical significance unknown.

TABLE 60: Dosing of antimicrobial agents for Patients with Chronic Kidney Disease (CKD) or End-Stage Renal Disease (ESRD).

Drug, dosing category	Dosage	
Sofosbuvir- Ledipasvir		
Cr CL > 30 ml/min	Usual dose: Sofosbuvir 400mg/Ledipasvir 90mg po once-daily	
Cr CL < 30 ml/min	Dose not established. Ledipasvir concentrations unlikely to be affected. Significant increase in sofosbuvir metabolite. Clinical significance unknown.	
Sofosbuvir- Velpatasvir		
Cr CL > 30 ml/min	Usual dose: Sofosbuvir 400mg- Velpatasvir 100mg po once daily	
Cr CL < 30 ml/min	Dose not established. No change in velpatasvir concentrations. Significant increase in sofosbuvir metabolite. Clinical significance unknown.	
Sofosbuvir- Velpatasvir-Voxilaprevir		
Cr CL > 30 ml/min	Usual dose: Sofosbuvir 400mg- Velpatasvir 100mg-Voxilaprevir 100mg po once daily	
Cr CL < 30 ml/min	Dose not established. No change in velpatasvir and voxilaprevir concentrations. Significant increase in sofosbuvir metabolite. Clinical significance unknown.	
Stavudine		
Cr CL > 50 mL/min	30 mg po q12h	The FDA recommends a higher dose in patients who are ≥ 60 kg, but this is associated with higher rates of toxicities (peripheral neuropathy, mitochondria toxicity, lactic acidosis).
Cr CL 26–50 mL/min	15 mg po q12h	
Cr CL ≤ 25 mL/min	15 mg po q24h	
Receiving hemodialysis	15 mg po q24h	
Receiving peritoneal dialysis	No data. Dose reduction recommended.	
Streptomycin		
Cr CL > 60 mL/min	MDRTB: 15 mg/kg IM q24h OR 25 mg/kg IM TIW	
Cr CL < 60 mL/min	Use with caution. Adjust dose based on concentrations. Target trough < 10 mcg/mL	
Sulfadiazine		
Cr CL > 50 mL/min	Usual dosage: 1-1.5 gm po q6h (1.5g for >60kg)	
Cr CL 10-50 mL/min	1-1.5 gm po q12h	
Cr CL < 10 mL/min; HD	1-1.5 gm po q24h	
Tenofovir alafenamide		
Cr CL ≥ 15 mL/min	25 mg po q24h. 92% higher tenofovir concentrations with CrCL 15-29ml/min (Custodio JM et al. AAC 2016).	
Cr CL < 15 mL/min	Avoid, but clinical significance unknown.	
Tenofovir alafenamide + emtricitabine		
Cr CL ≥ 30 mL/min	TAF/FTC 25/200 mg tab once daily	
Cr CL < 30 mL/min	Avoid co-formulation.	
Tenofovir DF		
Cr CL ≥ 50 mL/min	300 mg po q24h	
Cr CL 30–49 mL/min	300 mg po q48h. Consider switch to TAF.	

TABLE 60: Dosing of antimicrobial agents for Patients with Chronic Kidney Disease (CKD) or End-Stage Renal Disease (ESRD).

Drug, dosing category	Dosage
Tenofovir DF (cont.)	
Cr CL 10–29 mL/min	300 mg po q72-96h. Consider switch to TAF
Receiving hemodialysis	300 mg po every 7 days (an additional dose may be needed if >12h HD per week)
Receiving peritoneal dialysis	Receiving peritoneal dialysis
Tenofovir DF/Emtricitabine	
Cr CL ≥ 50 mL/min	300 /200 mg po q24h
Cr CL 30–49 mL/min	300/200 mg po q48h. Consider switch to TAF co-formulation
Cr CL < 30 mL/min	Coformulation not recommended. See TAF, TDF and FTC dosing recs.
Tenofovir DF/Lamivudine	**Avoid co-formulation with CrCL <50 ml.min**
Trimethoprim	
Cr CL > 30 mL/min	Usual dosage (mild to moderate PCP treatment): 5 mg/kg po q6–8h (in combination with dapsone)
Cr CL 10–30 mL/min	5 mg per kg po q12h (in combination with dapsone)
Cr CL < 10 mL/min	5 mg per kg po q24h (in combination with dapsone)
Trimethoprim-sulfamethoxazole	**PCP prophylaxis**
Cr CL > 30 mL/min	Usual dosage (PCP prophylaxis): 1 double strength dose po q24h; 1 double strength dose po 3 times per week; 1 single strength dose po q24h
Cr CL 15–30 mL/min	1/2 dose
Cr CL < 15 mL/min	1/2 dose
Trimethoprim-sulfamethoxazole	**PCP treatment**
Cr CL > 30 mL/min	Usual dosage (PCP treatment): 5 mg/kg (as TMP component) IV or po q6–8h
Cr CL 10–30 mL/min	5 mg per kg IV or po (as TMP component) q12h
Cr CL < 10 mL/min	5 mg per kg IV or po (as TMP component) q24h
Valacyclovir	
Cr CL > 50 mL/min	Usual dosage: 500 mg–1g po q8h
Cr CL 30-49 mL/min	500 mg–1g po q12h
Cr CL 10-20 mL/min	500-1 g mg po q24h
Cr CL < 10 mL/min	500 mg po q24h
Valganciclovir	
Cr CL > 50 mL/min	Usual dosage: 900 mg po q12h (induction); 900 mg po q24h (maintenance)
Cr CL 40–59 mL/min	450 mg q12h (induction); 450 mg q24h (maintenance).
Cr CL 25–39 mL/min	450 mg q.d.(induction); 450 mg q48h (maintenance)
Cr CL 10–24 mL/min	450 mg q48h (induction); 450 mg twice per week (maintenance).
Cr CL < 10 mL/min	Not recommended by US manufacturer. Use IV ganciclovir or consider 200 mg suspension TIW (induction)/ 100 mg suspension TIW (maintenance).
Receiving hemodialysis	Consider 200 mg oral powder formulation TIW (induction); 100 mg TIW (maintenance)

TABLE 60: Dosing of antimicrobial agents for Patients with Chronic Kidney Disease (CKD) or End-Stage Renal Disease (ESRD).

Drug, dosing category	Dosage
Voriconazole	
Cr CL > 50 ml/min	Aspergillosis: 6 mg/kg IV q12h x 2 (load), then 4 mg/kg q12h. Target trough > 2.05 mcg/mL Candidemia: 6 mg/kg IV q12h x 2 (load), then 3 mg/kg IV q12h Oral once clinically stable: 200–300 mg po q12h
Cr CL < 50 mL/min	Usual oral dose Avoid IV voriconazole because of potential toxicity due to accumulation of sulfobutylether-cyclodexrin (vehicle of IV product). Based on observational study this appears to be not a genuine concern.
Zidovudine	
Cr CL > 15 mL/min	Usual dose: 300 mg po q12h
Cr CL < 15 mL/min, HD, or PD	100 mg po q8h or 300 mg po q24h

NOTES

CPSIA information can be obtained
at www.ICGtesting.com
Printed in the USA
LVHW072353130721
692558LV00008B/339